D0783756

6/2281218

VOGUE
make-up

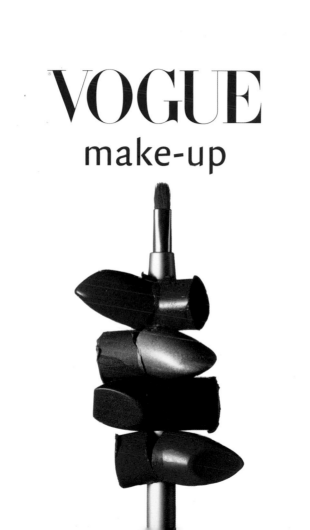

THIS IS A CARLTON BOOK

The Vogue logo is a registered trademark
of Condé Nast Publications Limited
Photographs copyright © 2001 Condé Nast
Publications Limited
Text copyright © 2001 Juliet Cohen
Design copyright © 2001 Carlton Books Limited

First published in 2001
This edition published in 2009 by
Carlton Books Limited
20 Mortimer Street
London W1T 3JW

All rights reserved
A CIP catalogue record for this book is available
from the British Library
ISBN 978 1 84442 102 2

Printed and bound in Dubai

The author and publisher have made every effort to
ensure that all information is correct and up to date
at the time of publication. Neither the author nor the
publisher can accept responsibility for any accident,
injury or damage that results from using the ideas,
information or advice offered in this book.

The application and quality of beauty products, beauty
treatments, herbal preparations and essential oils is
beyond the control of the above parties, who cannot be
held responsible for any problems resulting from their
use. Always follow the manufacturer's instructions and
if in doubt, seek further advice.

Do not use herbal preparations or essential oils
without prior consultation with a qualified practitioner
or medical doctor if you are pregnant, taking any form
of medication, or if you suffer from oversensitive skin.

VOGUE
make-up

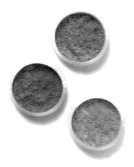

Juliet Cohen

CARLTON
BOOKS
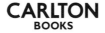

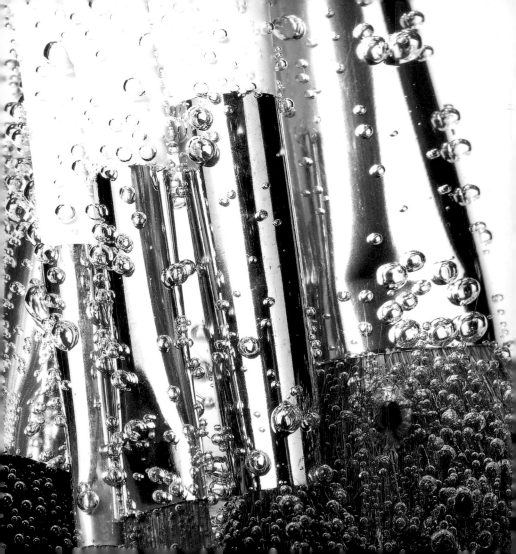

contents

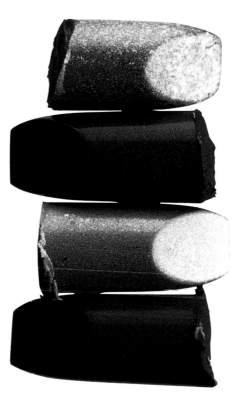

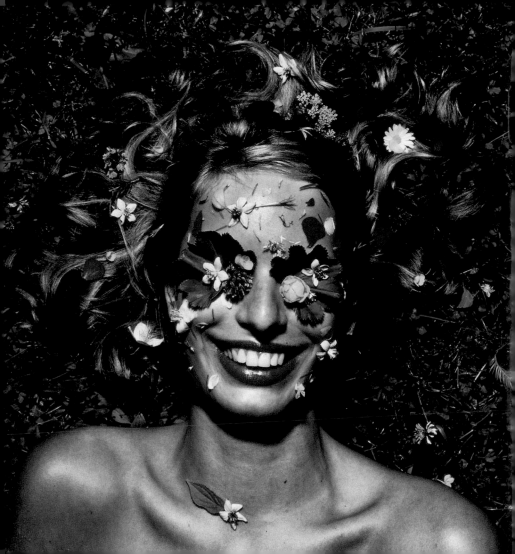

introduction

When I left university, I was lucky enough to land a job at the publishers Condé Nast, working in the beauty department of a busy magazine. It was there, as part of my work experience, that my eyes were first opened to the magic world that is make-up. Nestled inside the enormous beauty cupboard, I spent hours dabbling with glittery powders, shimmering creams and glistening lotions. For the first time in my life, it struck me that make-up gives every woman the potential to be beautiful. Not because I believe you need to disguise yourself to look great, but more because I think you need to feel great to look it, and playing with the magic dust of make-up makes you feel just that.

The technicolour world of colour cosmetics offers every woman unlimited possibilities, and some of the greatest female icons of our time are chameleons, changing their entire look as often as designers change their hemlines. Think Kate Moss, the late Diana, Princess of Wales, Gwyneth Paltrow and Madonna, to name but a few. Each share the courage to experiment, and they all have power – power derived from understanding which tools are at their fingertips, and using them to their best advantage.

This book is not about rigid rules and instructions, nor is it a bible of the best lipsticks or face creams: because the bottom line is that there is no ultimate product. The right lipstick is simply the one that you choose to wear right now. Of course, with cosmetic counters groaning under the weight of a whole universe of colour and texture, actually deciding what you want to wear is far from easy. Which might explain why so many women are actually afraid of make-up – afraid to experiment with anything new, and above all, afraid of colour. This is an attempt to allay some of those fears, and demystify some fundamental techniques.

Thanks to many of the wonderful make-up artists, models and scientific researchers whom I have had the privilege of working with, *Vogue Make-up* is packed with insider tips and information. Of course the *Vogue* reader is intelligent enough to make her own decisions, and tailor her cosmetics to suit her individual needs. The advice offered in these pages is simply intended to make you question why you want to achieve a certain look, and then help you go about attaining it.

Of course, the subject matter in itself is not new – make-up is as old as the universe, so to put the present in perspective, I have started with a condensed view of the past. The history of make-up fascinates me, and I hope that it interests you. To make things easy, *Vogue Make-up* is broken down into sections: skincare, face shape and skin tone, tools of the trade, foundation, eyes, lips, cheeks, body and hair make-up, and hands and feet are all dealt with. I hope that there is something here that appeals to readers of every age group and every background. Because what differentiates our vision of beauty today from the way we saw it yesterday is that today's beauty is inclusive – you no longer need to conform to look great, you just need to look like you.

I hope that you enjoy reading *Vogue Make-up* as much as I have enjoyed writing it.

what is beauty?

'A witty woman is a treasure;
a witty beauty is a power.'
George Meredith, poet

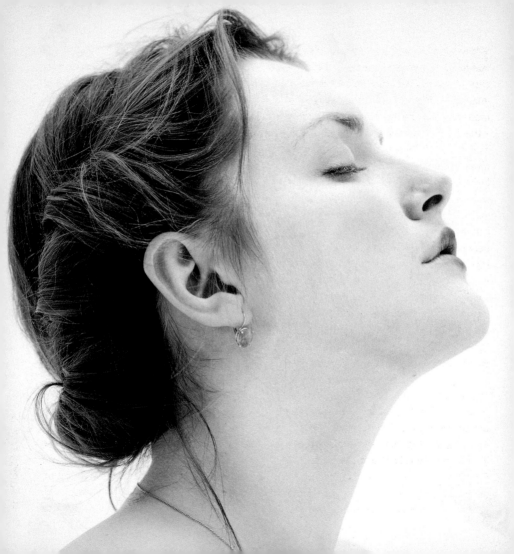

Beauty is like a magnet – it attracts others to it. Yet while elements of beauty are easy to spot, what truly defines it remains intangible. This is because in today's post-modern world, beauty is about individuality – there are no norms, and no given ideals to aspire to. Of course, this makes beauty a more democratic commodity than ever before, but it also creates a dichotomy – today's beauty must possess two types of allure: the internal and the external. While external beauty is largely reliant on other people's judgement (an accepted beauty is lent her standing by those around her), internal beauty is something we all possess, something that makes us stand out from the crowd, and that by proxy affects our physical appearance as well as our mental outlook. Rather like the chicken and the egg, if you feel your best, you usually look it, and vice versa.

The power of beauty is immeasurable. Delve back into your deepest memories – why was the prettiest girl at school always popular? And why was the man with the scarred face always stereotyped as the movie's baddie? As far back as ancient civilizations, physical perfection was revered as a gift from the gods, while physical deformity, the 'outer display of inner corruption', was castigated. Although society has moved on a long way since then, make-up as a way of attaining beauty is still a powerful tool. Even the most exquisite face is improved with make-up – hence the late Diana, Princess of Wales, came to *Vogue* for a restyle; many a supermodel will only agree to be photographed if she can have her favourite make-up artist in tow; celebrities demand final approval of pictures before publication; and politician after politician improves his look to try to increase his votes. Hardly an American president in living memory has resisted the odd nip or tuck, or at least a set of pearly-white improvements to his winning smile.

Of course, beautifying yourself has a superficial aspect, but it has a deeper psychological one, too. I firmly believe that if you look and feel your best you approach day-to-day life in a totally different manner – quite literally with your head up. Indeed, it is a scientifically proven fact that those who are happy with their appearance perform better, and those who perform achieve. So any way in which we can cosmetically enhance the canvas nature gave us is a bonus, and bit by bit, decade by decade, make-up has contributed to our idea of ourselves. In the twentieth century alone, the 1920s vamp dabbled with beauty spots, the 1950s starlet wore glossy lips and glamorous lashes and the 1970s disco queen lit up a party as much as a disco ball. By the 1990s, of course, technology had orbited beyond the realms of the familiar, and a plethora of textures, tones and colours became readily available right through from one end of the market to the other. Hence the beauty business, once a basic cold-cream/panstick/coral-or-red-lipstick business, is now a billion-dollar global industry.

This infinite choice, combined with changing demographics (the growing numbers of interracial partnerships is quite literally changing the face of humanity), are to be thanked for the twenty-first century's increasing freedom. Our accepted ideas of beauty are being forced to change, as it becomes physically impossible to conform to any one type. We now stand poised on the threshold of a whole new era – one in which everybody can be beautiful, and the ideal is simply an individual's potential fulfilled.

In an age when we can remove unwanted hair permanently and painlessly, prevent premature skin ageing and thus turn back the clock, achieve year-round colour without exposing ourselves to a single harmful ray of sun, make our short hair long overnight, enjoy the permanent arched eyebrows nature never gave us, and contour our faces and bodies with relative ease, we really can be exactly who we want to be. Throwing off the shackles of conformity does not mean we need to care less, however; it means we must care more.

Firstly, we have a responsibility to enjoy looking good: make-up is meant to be fun, after all. If you put aside the time to dabble with glossy compacts, shimmery powders and creamy potions, you actually allow yourself to take time out of a hectic schedule, and concentrate on yourself alone. A few such minutes of relaxation, stolen like this on a daily basis, are healthier for mind and body than a full hour's massage taken only once a month. And as we all know, a healthy mind (the start of 'inner beauty') means a healthy body (the start of 'outer beauty').

To attain the 'inner' half of the beauty package, we must face the new century with a new attitude to lifestyle – one that incorporates healthy living, healthy eating and a sensible commitment to exercise. Time is one of the most valuable commodities in the modern world – if you invest your time wisely now, you will reap the benefits of mental health and physical strength in the future. With a healthy outlook assured, the gloss and the glamour are there for the taking. The difficulty that the modern woman faces is the confusion of choice – exactly which option should I take? Remember that glossy magazines are there to suggest, no longer to dictate, and whether you leaf through Vogue to lift a look entirely, or to borrow some ideas and expand on others, is up to you. A beautiful woman in today's world is one who is happy with her own identity – not one who looks as though she has been tortured and squeezed into somebody else's.

Above all else, 'We have freedom of style now,' says make-up guru Vincent Longo. 'There are so many timeless beauty looks and so many beauty icons. It doesn't really matter which you choose. Modern beauty is about enhancing your own features and looking pretty and approachable.'

The point of democratic beauty is to enjoy it, and that holds for twenty-first-century man.

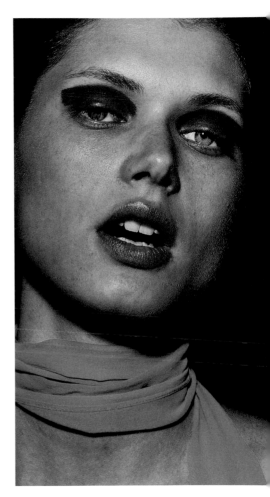

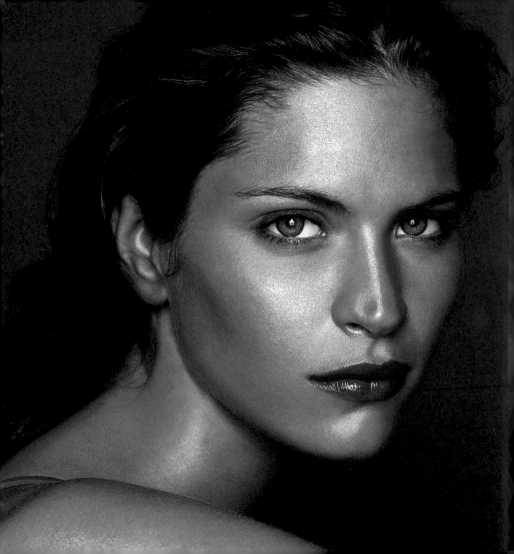

With women's choices now infinite, men are pushing the boundaries, too. While anything more than a shave or a haircut was once a statement of sexual preference, today's men are free to explore. No longer obliged to dabble secretly in their girlfriend's bathroom cupboard, millennium man indulges in facials, body masks, manicures (with polish), and even waxing and cosmetic surgery. And why should men not enjoy it? In ancient times any bloke with an ounce of self-esteem took regular saunas, pushed back his cuticles, made sure his hair was perfect and applied cosmetics to enhance his features. What seems 'right' is simply what we are used to, after all: think of the (traditional) Englishman who scoffs at wearing fragrance, when no Frenchman worth his onions would be smelled without it. Many major companies have now launched lines of 'make-up for men', with foundation – or 'concealer' in male cosmetics' vocabulary – leading the way.

The rapidly expanding consumer market owes a debt of gratitude to technology. With the Internet revolution and arrival of e-commerce, we are now able to buy everything from Brylcreem to body paint from the comfort of home. Thanks to virtual technology, we can already download our image at our work-station, try out different hair colours and make-up on screen, and decide exactly which products to use for real. Before long we will also be able to download 3-D images, and even smell and touch, making drastic haircuts, unfortunate scent and make-up choices, and even surgical faux pas things of the past.

I do not advocate a society where self-esteem is based solely on looks (woe betide any of us if we create a world of Dorian Grays ready to sacrifice all in the quest for beauty), but I do believe that looking good makes you feel better, and if it makes you feel better, then do it. Looking breathtaking is no longer a happy accident of birth – you can look stunning whatever your genetic make-up. While the quest for beauty can sometimes be frustrating, for the most part it is a lot of fun, and ultimately empowering.

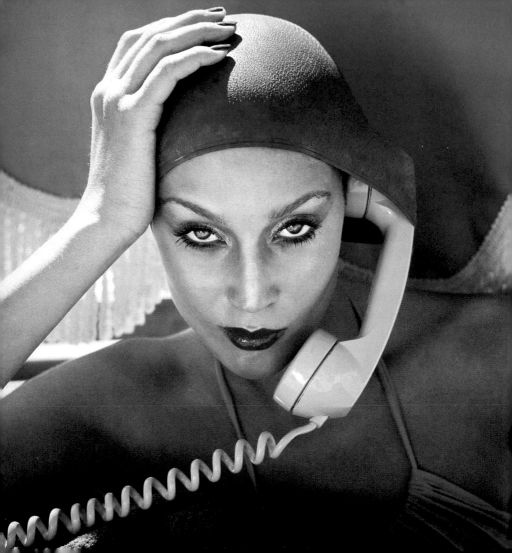

twenty-first century beauty

21

'I am constantly amazed by the technology. It is giving us so much choice and freedom.'

Terry de Gunzburg, make-up artist

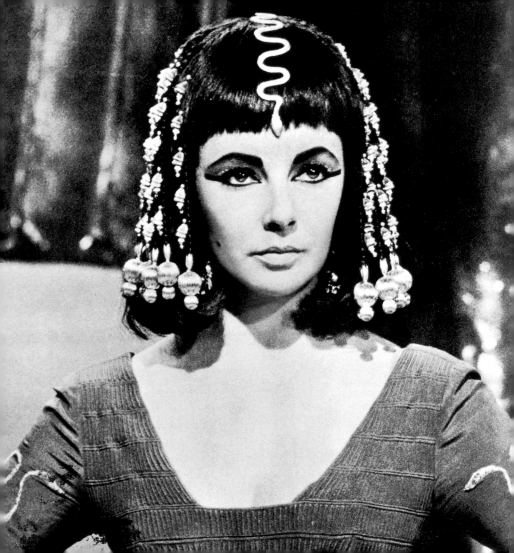

ANCIENT CIVILIZATIONS

The pursuit of beauty is no modern phenomenon – many ancient civilizations considered beauty a gift from the gods, and as such it brought influence and power. No other people were more obsessed by appearance than the ancient Greeks, whose entire culture revolved around the worship of the ultimate human form. Men even more than women dedicated their whole lives to achieving physical perfection – even if it killed them. For while the fashionable white face paint sported by the upper classes was made of poisonous lead, those who were literally dying to remove unwanted hair used orpiment (a derivative of arsenic) to make a depilatory.

There is hardly an item of make-up or a cosmetic treatment that exists today that was not first used in ancient Egypt. As far back as 10,000 bc both men and women were sprinkling themselves with deliciously scented oils, and using paint and coloured powders to enhance their features. They rouged their lips and cheeks, painted their hands and feet with henna, traced the veins on their breasts with blue dye, and shone out at festivities with gold painted nipples. The kohl-eyed look (reinvented for the modern world by Mary Quant in the 1960s) was originally the trademark of Cleopatra.

The beauty business is as old as humanity – a proper cosmetics industry was in full swing by the time of the Pharaohs. Cosmetics makers (often priests) would obtain mined chunks of coloured pigment, then sell it in palettes that Shu Uemura would be proud of. Yellow and orange ochre was used as face paint, while green eyeshadow (made of verdigris and resin) was a favourite eye opener. Powders and pastes were sold in tubes or jars and, just like today, women would gather around cosmetics counters eager to try out new products. Being beautiful has never come cheap – high prices were asked for nut- and almond-oil skincare lotions, hair dye made of cow's blood and tortoiseshell, and mirrors made of polished metals. This made cosmetics the privilege (and thus also the outward sign) of the upper classes. Only the highest echelon society could indulge in face creams made of

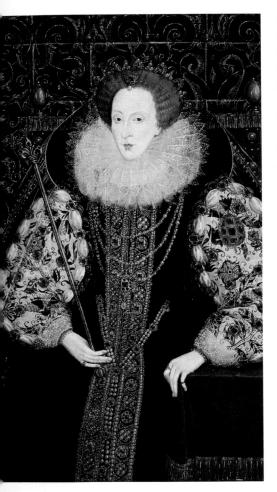

bullock's bile and ostrich eggs, masks produced from crocodile excrement and wrinkle creams made from genital extracts. No wonder they were so keen that these treasures accompany them in the afterlife.

Such delicacies were not confined to one continent alone. The Assyrians equalled anything the Egyptians had to offer when it came to cosmetic enhancement. Curling tongs, metal orange sticks and pumice stones were in plentiful supply, in Babylonia as well as Persia. And it didn't stop there. Throughout history, men and women have cosmetically enhanced their features (often at the expense of their health) to attract the opposite sex and court power. Elizabethan courtiers, for example, used arsenic as a type of face whitener (a pale complexion proving you were wealthy enough to stay indoors, a tan being the obvious result of outdoor labour). Far away in Africa, tribal warriors traditionally used both face and body paint as signals to the gods, to bring them health and prosperity or make them fertile.

1920s and 1930s

By the more puritan late Victorian era make-up had gone underground, rearing its head only as the trademark of a stripper or a whore. By the 1920s, however, young women had tired of this colourless existence, and make-up staged a comeback – putting on lipstick was soon to become the gesture of the decade. At this point conformity was everything: in the quest for the perfect English rose complexion, women on both sides of the Atlantic had treatments to bleach their skin, and splashed out on copious amounts of rouge and talcum powder to create what nature had denied them. Even those who resisted lipstick and rouge succumbed to lightening their skin with face powder. In Europe the battle against ageing had begun – women in Paris and London were having face-lifts long before they became popular in the USA. While the English were (secretly) undergoing the knife, their American counterparts were settling for skin conditioning of a less radical variety: sales of Pond's Cold Cream were rocketing, along with more sophisticated remedies by Helena Rubinstein and Elizabeth Arden.

While polite society recoiled in horror at the onslaught of eyebrow pencils, eyeshadow, mascara, blusher, lip pencils and rouge, younger women revelled in it. Now that painted nails no longer signified a 'painted woman', blood red became the colour of the decade. On every street corner beauty salons popped up, offering massages, manicures, facials, hair colouring and makeovers. The banner of respectability was the salons' best advertisement, and before long treatments were so popular that there were waiting lists for appointments. In addition, the universal use of make-up brought with it new dilemmas surrounding etiquette. Even the most well-bred women could now be caught brushing their hair at the table, or leaving lipstick smears on napkins. Beauty editors were swift with their advice: put yourself together before you go out, and leave yourself alone in public. DIY beauty thrived just as much, and every department store had huge cosmetics counters. By 1925 it was estimated that American women alone spent $1 billion on beauty products. Once, wearing make-up meant painting a questionable moral picture; now no girl worth her lipstick would be seen without it.

The Depression of the 1930s did nothing to curb women's addiction to cosmetics. Like children let loose in a fantasy land, they revelled in the choice of colour – a whole spectrum away from the mundane reality of their everyday existence. With green, blue and lilac coming out of Paris, the idea of wearing make-up to match your clothes and not your skin tone was born. Thanks to the genius of Coco Chanel, make-up houses that had already raked in fortunes from their alabaster powders now made more money selling bronzers. The healthy outdoor look soon replaced the porcelain complexions of the fickle followers of fashion. Beauty was no longer left to fate, as nearly every woman now possessed a plethora of make-up products, along with eyelash curlers, false lashes and a regular appointment with a hairdresser. Of course, exploitation touched men as well as women: once beards were deemed unfashionable, beauty houses reaped the benefits of increased sales of razors, lathers, creams and colognes.

This was the decade when Yardley opened a shop in London and Max Factor launched its legendary panstick. The 1930s' most defining beauty characteristic, however, was the Hollywood star, icons like Gloria Swanson and Greta Garbo, offering glamorous escapism from the humdrum reality of Depression. Every woman wanted to look like a star, and if she could not actually be Marlene Dietrich she could, at least, wear products called Starlet Shadow and Cinema Sable.

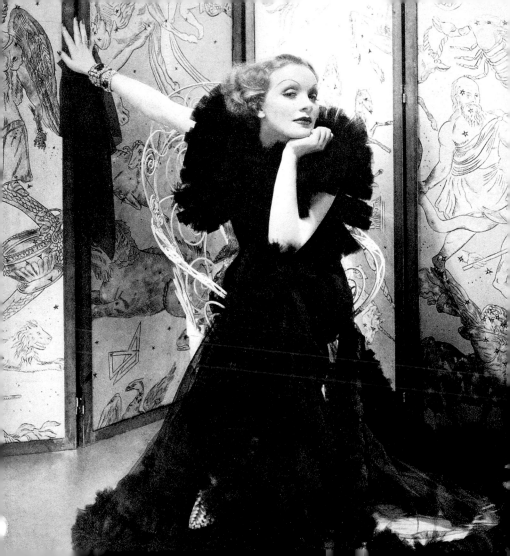

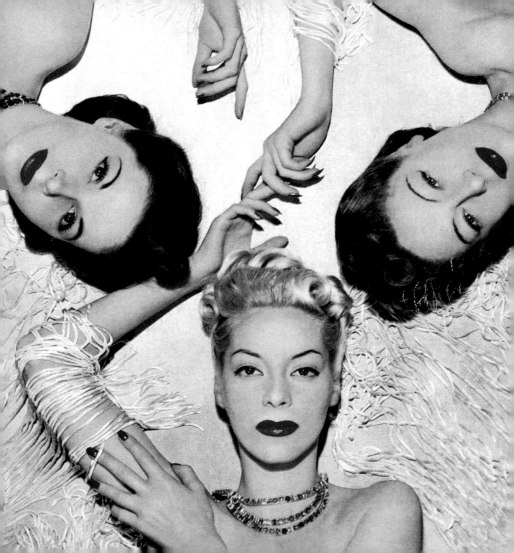

1940s and 1950s

Escapism was also the byword of the 1940s. While the onset of war threatened to deal a hard blow to the cosmetics industry (short supplies entailed limited alcohol for perfume, reduced supplies of fats for lipsticks, and little or no plastic for packaging), women's attachment to make-up increased. With the conscription in the war years of single females aged between 18 and 25, imagination and initiative were key to survival; although rations could curb a woman's spending, they served only to increase her vanity. When stockings proved impossible to come by, leg make-up provided the perfect answer – seams pencilled in with eyeliner became so common that they were almost fashionable, and body make-up caught on. The sale of men's products soared, too – the great morale boost of luxury products meant that scents for men and soap in 'man-sized bars' became number one gifts for servicemen. Even those who would balk at the mention of 'face powder' were happy to cover themselves in talc. The American influence hit Europe big time – the presence of American GIs (with their gifts of nylon stockings) added a thrill of excitement to an otherwise tense and worrying time. Hollywood was still the biggest influence on beauty, with Bette Davis, Lauren Bacall and Rita Hayworth as memorable icons.

Glamour, glamour, glamour was the mantra of the 1950s, as the end of the war signalled the beginning of a whole new era. Dior's New Look revolutionized the world of fashion, with models on the Paris runways boasting pinched-in waists and sculpted busts. This overtly feminine look was accompanied by unashamedly made-up faces and the resumed supply of cosmetics meant that women would make the most of it; eye make-up became a special focus, with false lashes, plenty of shadow and liner, and lashings of lengthening mascara. Now that the grey war years were over, blue, green and violet shadow signalled the

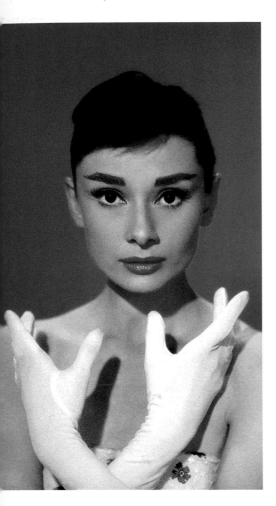

embrace of a whole new world of technicolour luxury. Short haircuts were a form of liberation for women, everyone reeked of violets, and Coty, Rimmel and Charles of the Ritz became big names in the world of make-up. Revlon put cosmetics truly on the fashion map – thanks to Charles Revson, a new shade of lipstick and nail varnish would now be launched at six-month intervals instead of once a year. This gave women more choice than ever before, a phenomenon reflected by the differing icons of the era: while Grace Kelly, Vivien Leigh, Jane Russell and Marilyn Monroe offered womanly beauty on the one hand, Audrey Hepburn introduced gamine chic on the other.

1960s

The birth of the 1960s signalled a decade of rebellion. The Pill, the Beatles and the youthful social revolution meant that teenagers finally had a voice. No longer content to look like their mothers, English girls saw Twiggy as the epitome of a whole new look. Goodbye hourglass figures (throw out your 'roll-ons' and your 'waspies'), hello small bottoms and skinny legs. This was a landmark in defining the new female shape: women no longer felt trapped by their underwear. To accompany this freedom came the introduction of pretty knickers, unpadded bras and tights.

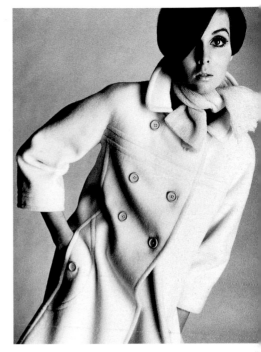

Sixties' girls quite literally let their hair down. The formal styles of the 1950s were replaced by long, straight locks, a Vidal Sassoon 'bob' or detachable hairpieces and ponytails. The babydoll look, miniskirts and knee-high boots, formed the basis of a new uniform (the young didn't want to look like their parents but they did want to look like each other). Now that the baby-boomers had come of age, a generation of disposable income became available. (Estée Lauder cashed in on this with a nail varnish called 24K gold, which was made of exactly that.)

Make-up provided as good a badge of membership of the new-minted social group as miniskirts: kohl-lined eyelids and blue eyeshadow (courtesy of Mary Quant) greeted you on every street corner, and false lashes – and even eyebrows – lent everybody the same defined curves and exaggerated eye sockets. Blusher (the new name for rouge) was big news in the 1960s. Every shade from pink to pearl was available in washes, creams and cakes of colour. These were blended into the hairline, under the chin and on to the neck – the creation of a healthy, outdoor look was of the essence.

Food for skin became food for thought in this decade. For the first time skin was given independent status as the starting point for make-up. High-protein skin treats included ingredients such as honey, royal jelly, vitamins and minerals; bestsellers were Innoxa's Living Peach face cream, and Lentheric's Special Formula Skin Food. It wasn't just topical nourishers that were given the 'good enough to eat' treatment: flavoured lipsticks and roll-on glosses in cola, cherry or strawberry also made great headway on the make-up front.

Now that colour cosmetics were as sophisticated as they were popular, the professional make-up artist came into being. Not just an advisor to the business but also a mouthpiece for the public, an Italian nobleman, the make-up artist Pablo (with his staple colours of mauve and pistachio), won Elizabeth Arden much-coveted press attention.

Men enjoyed the cultural revolution, too, with males spending fortunes on tinting their eyebrows and as their hair grew longer and wider, having body waves and blow-dries. Twiggy, Catherine Deneuve, Natalie Wood and Bridget Bardot were the icons of the decade.

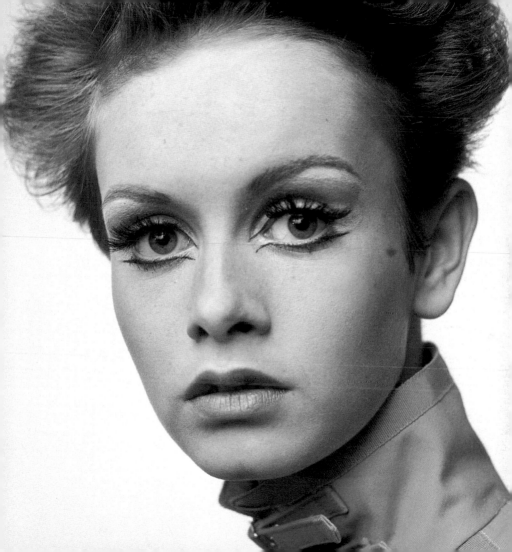

1970s

Sex, drugs, rock'n'roll; the devalued pound; war in Vietnam; the assasination of Kennedy: all these were part of the rich background that gave its character to the 1970s. After ten years of community feeling among young people, the world economic downturn led to disappointment and the desire for an alternative society. Freedom and

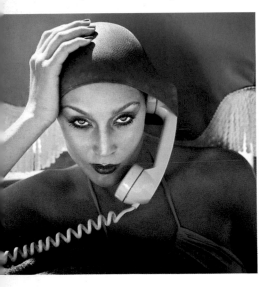

self-expression were paramount to the disillusioned youth, whose permissive attitude permeated every aspect of their lifestyle. The total breakdown of traditional values led to the upsurge of the hippie lifestyle, and many set up communes where drugs and sex were readily available. At the same time the disco scene exploded, with glittery eye make-up, platform shoes and Afro hairdos lighting up the dance floors.

With every rule rejected, men and women left more to nature. This was reflected not only in their clothes but in their physical appearance, too. The scruffy look hit big time – hair was long and natural, beards were back, and many women gave up on depilation.

Feminism was taken up in earnest during the 1970s. The launch of *Cosmopolitan* magazine, with its revolutionary discussion of orgasms, and Germaine Greer's *The Female Eunuch*, struck a chord with women on both sides of the Atlantic. Even James Bond was caught wrestling with female opponents...

In spite of this, advertising imagery was, on the whole, nostalgic. Girls with long flowing tresses, in turn-of-the-century clothing filled television space as well as billboards, and companies like Yardley and Cadbury's (with its famous Flake advert), benefitted from this atmospheric escapism.

Artifice was superseded by the natural – fruit-flavoured roll-on lip gloss and face creams packed with natural ingredients such as rose, avocado, yogurt and honey were cult items. For the first time ever, anything 'green' was cool; vegetarianism, no longer considered faddish or outlandish, filtered into mainstream diets. Estée Lauder launched Clinique, with its three-step cleanse, tone and moisturize routine, and women went wild about skincare. Goldie Hawn, Bo Derek and Farrah Fawcett were the beauties whom women aspired to look like, with their fresh-faced, clean-haired, uncontrived look.

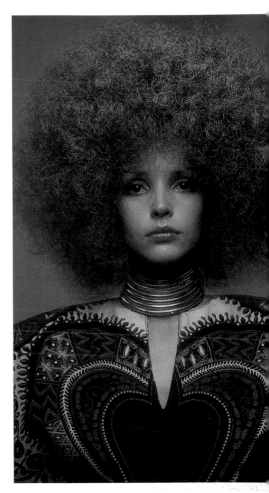

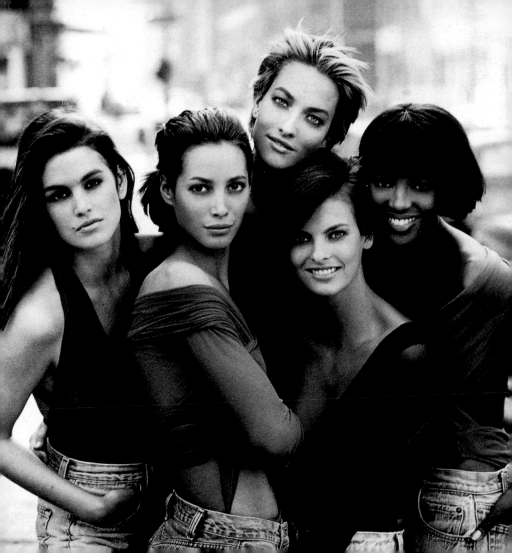

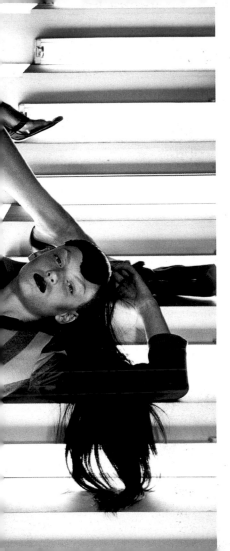

granted recognition, and women began to realize that they did not need to emulate Cindy Crawford to look great.

This rejection of conformity was reflected in the beauty world: unisex fragrances such as CK One became cult items, and the phrase 'no-make-up make-up' was coined. Women wanted to look good naturally, and with the arrival of cult brand MAC and 'make-up artists' make-up' there was a move away from traditional products. Bobbi Brown, Vincent Longo and François Nars were revered as the new major players. Huge scientific breakthroughs were happening in skincare, and consumer expectations increased accordingly. Even high-street brands began to incorporate new technology in their products.

The 1990s saw England make a bold mark on the global fashion map. John Galliano and Alexander McQueen designed for French fashion houses, London became the place to be and Britain was 'Cool Britannia'.

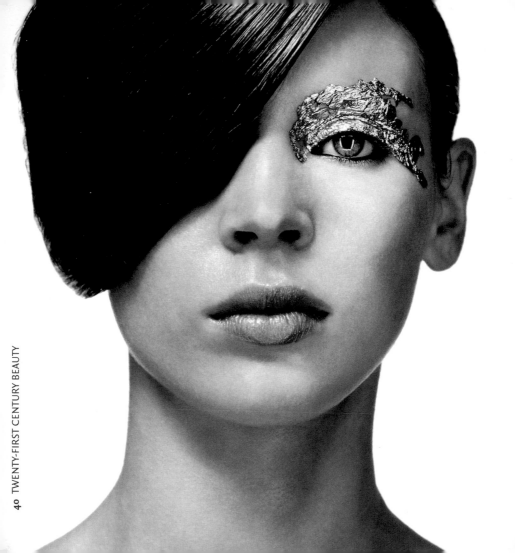

2000 and the future

Choice and individuality promise to be the buzzwords of twenty-first-century beauty. Thanks to technological breakthroughs in skincare and make-up that nobody would have thought possible just a decade ago, we are constantly pushing new boundaries. Whereas once the choice of colour signalled consumer freedom, today's woman wants an active involvement in the texture of her make-up, too. No longer content with five shades of foundation, we want hundreds, and we want them in every finish from satin to gloss to matt to light-responsive to light-reflective, and so on. Whatever our ethnicity, we refuse to be pigeonholed; it is no longer sufficient just to have 'pink tones' or 'yellow'. The old rule book was too simplistic, and we do not care for the rules now anyway.

Twenty-first-century make-up will carve a couture route, with people asserting their individuality by buying custom-blend products in everything from make-up to haircare to skincare to fragrance. Body jewellery and adornment will become more mainstream,

too. The multipurpose product (take François Nars's marvellous Multiple stick, which can be used anywhere from face to arms to décolletage) gives us another pointer in the direction of future make-up. More and more products will go the multi-function route, with day and night creams being dispensed from one bottle (suncream packaging is already going this way), and fragrance that will treat your skin – and even bleach it – as well as enhance your mood. Ease and versatility will be key to most women, as we travel more, and want to travel light.

With breakthroughs in modern medicine promising to extend our lifespans radically, the youth culture that exists today will change. As our life expectancy increases, society will have to cater for a growing sector of aged people, and so our very definition of what is old will change. More revolutions in laser and cosmetic surgery are just around the corner, and while we will all want to reach a ripe old age we will certainly not want to look it.

The holistic lifestyle will be central to twenty-first-century beauty. People will take care of their spiritual as well as their physical wellbeing, and most of us will service our bodies just as we now service our cars. More 'outlandish' treatments will become the norm, as travel makes the riches of cultures and customs across the globe accessible, and men will spend more time pampering themselves. Cosmetics for males will steadily lose their taboo, as companies invest more time and money developing make-up for men – a natural progression from an already awakened interest in skincare. In fact, the UK is now the fastest-growing European market for male toiletries, with teenage boys (influenced by the rise of boy bands) a new target audience.

Thanks to technology and to a rapidly expanding spectrum of colour and texture, make-up has progressed from fashion in a way it never could have previously. For the first time in history the beauty industry will set the trends for fashion folk to follow, and this, above all else, is what promises to be the biggest breakthrough for twenty-first-century beauty.

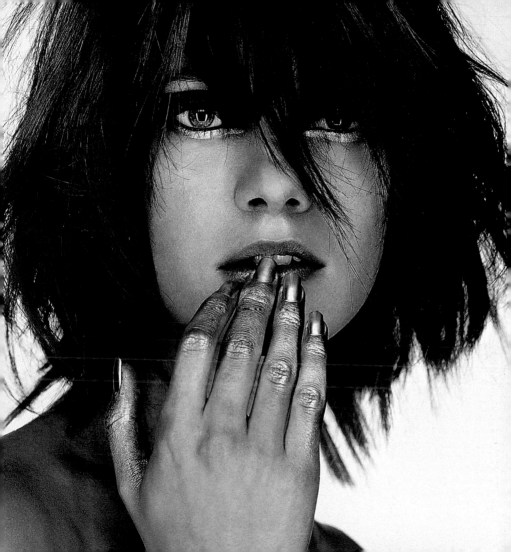

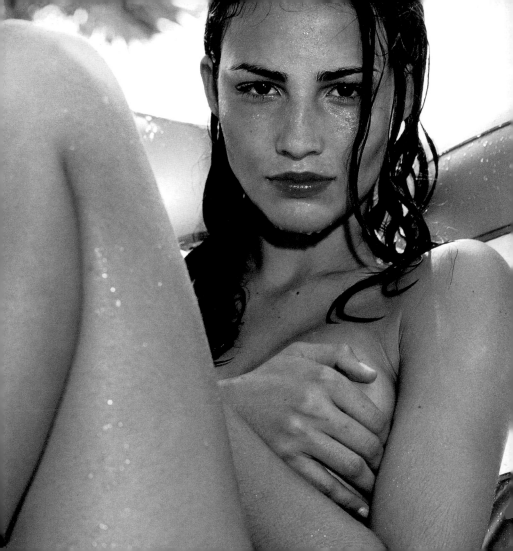

1

skin

'Achieving the appearance of radiant and truly
healthy skin is always a goal for me. I feel
prettiest when I am confident about my skin.'
Christy Turlington, supermodel

Think of your skin as an artist's canvas – without a smooth one, no amount of make-up will help create a masterpiece. However, thanks to the revolution in skincare technology at the end of the twentieth century, you no longer have to be born with perfect skin to reap its benefits. In fact, the thinking behind modern skincare is so advanced that discoveries in both texture and formulation are now used routinely to enhance make-up, haircare and suncreams.

The skin is our largest organ – if you slipped it off and popped it on the scales it would weigh approximately 2.75 kg (6 lbs). It protects our insides, acts as a vehicle of elimination to help excrete the body's toxic waste, and provides us with an in-built thermostat (we sweat when we feel hot, and increase our energy supplies by shivering when we feel cold). Most important of all, we do most of our breathing through our skin.

Because the skin is, to some extent, separated from the other vital organs, it is usually the first area to show signs of stress, which means that however great your skin is, you need to take care of it. While today's skincare is scientifically proven to help turn back the clock (thank you, retinoids), we do still find ourselves fighting a constant battle against skin ageing. When we are in our twenties and thirties our skin renews itself easily and efficiently (roughly every 28 days) because the horny layer is able to retain enough moisture to keep the epidermis fresh and the complexion smooth and refined. But as we get older, environmental factors such as dryness, ultraviolet exposure, oxidation and stress endanger both our skin's health and its

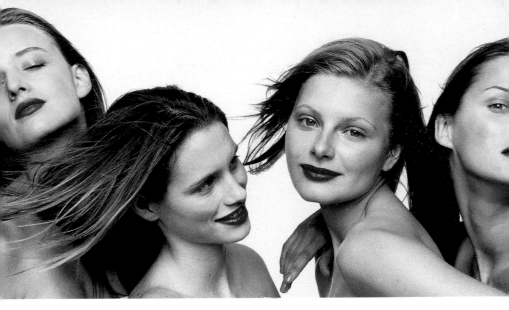

appearance. Because our skin is a living organism, its needs change according to condition and the climate. In the search for the Holy Grail of skin perfection, we must respect these differing needs, and treat our faces accordingly. Think of it as a kind of epidermal annuity – if you invest the time and effort now, you will reap the benefits every year of your future.

Sadly, there's no such thing as a miracle youth restorative, and while creams improve your skin's condition, nothing protects its future like a healthy lifestyle. George Orwell once said, 'At 50, everyone has the face he deserves.' So make sure you deserve a good one.

your skin type

DRY SKIN

Today the term 'skin type' is something of an anathema. We all know that our skin can change – from greasy one day to dry the next (depending on fluctuating hormones and outside factors like the weather), and that we need to change our skincare routine accordingly. While it is true that Mediterranean skin can be prone to greasiness, or an English rose complexion to sensitivity, remember that 'it ain't necessarily so ...'

If crocodile skin describes your face as well as your handbag, you probably have dry skin. While you do not suffer the acne angst of your oily counterparts, you are a walking advertisement for Old Mother Time. Dry skin tends to age quickly and can be flaky. Although its pores are barely visible, and sebum production is minimal, the idea that dry skin suffers no break-outs is a myth.

Most people try to combat dry skin by saturating it with oil – not the best plan if you realize that dry skin is actually thirsty. What it needs is a regular supply of water (taken internally) as well as a boost by using the right face creams.

Because we lose about 600 ml (1 pint) of body fluid a day through epidermal evaporation, those with dry skin should ensure that they drink at least eight glasses of water a day. In particular, air conditioning and wind exposure aggravate dry skin, so make sure you always wear a protective moisturizer. Cream cleansers are best for dry skin, as water-soluble products tend to exacerbate the problem. As well as moisturizing religiously twice a day, an occasional intensive night treatment will boost your daily routine (skin absorbs active ingredients best when you are asleep).

Choosing the right make-up is key to disguising dry skin: while powder products will stick in every crease and crevice and make your face look like a road map, oil-based products (with ingredients such as silicones) will glide on easily without cracking. Cream blushers are easy to apply with the fingertips, but if you don't want to look like Aunt Sally in a take from Worzel Gummidge, make sure that you blend, blend, blend.

OILY SKIN

You win the jackpot on the ageing lottery if you suffer from oily skin. But while the unsightly lines and wrinkles of premature ageing are kept at bay until later in life, oily skin presents its owner with something of a paradox. Both the best and the worst thing about this skin type (typical of those with olive complexions and Mediterranean features), is that it secretes a lot of sebum. On the one hand this natural moisturizer protects the epidermis from external aggressors

SKIN TYPE CHECKLIST

1 Does your skin feel tight and flaky? If so, it is probably dry. Remember that thirsty skin needs water, not oil, so drink plenty of water, and use moisturizers with a high water content.

2 Oily skin? Avoid harsh products that will strip the skin of oil and encourage flakiness. Instead, opt for an oil-based cleanser, which dissolves sebum, and moisturize with an oil-free lotion.

3 If you are unlucky enough to have genuinely sensitive skin, avoid products that contain known allergens such as fragrance, live plant extracts or lanolin.

such as climate change and central heating, and keeps it young and supple, but on the other hand it leaves the skin susceptible to seborrhoea (overproduction of oil) and the accompanying open pores, angry red spots and break-outs.

In the vigorous attempt to combat the notoriously greasy T-zone, those with oily complexions are prone to overwash and overstimulate the skin. Sadly, instead of minimizing the problem, this serves to increase it as the sebaceous glands work overtime to produce even more sebum to compensate. Avoid the temptation to use harsh strippers in the treatment of oily skin, for although products with a high alcohol content give a momentary sensation of freshness, they make it much worse in the long term.

Make-up choices are paramount, and if you do not want your beautifully painted face to slip down your chin and on to your cashmere sweater, you had better learn the meaning of some beauty jargon. Avoid, at all costs, products that claim to be 'satin finish' or 'glossy'. These contain fats and silicones that will slide around your face and end up looking greasy. Opt instead for 'oil-free' make-up and oil-free moisturizers to stay shine free. Avoid using foundation round the T-zone, and use powder blusher and eyeshadow that will not only stay put but also help absorb any excess oil to keep you feeling comfortable. While some cosmetics companies insist that cream cleansers are fine for oily skins, I find the wash-off type more helpful, as they leave you feeling squeaky clean, just like washing with soap and water.

COMBINATION SKIN

This is as near to 'normal' as any one skin type gets. Most of us, at some time or another, go through dry, sensitive and greasy stages, and sometimes even a combination of all three at once. Combination skins have a T-zone that is generally oilier than other areas, with the cheeks suffering from intermittent dryness. Sadly, nobody has yet invented a product that can successfully deliver oil to certain areas while absorbing it from others, so the best way to treat combination skin is to treat it in separate sections. Buying products for dry and oily skin may sound like a double outlay, but each product will last you twice as long, so think of it as an investment. Make-up choices are easier for combination skin, and really it is a question of a little of what you fancy does you good. Trial and error is the best method of both elimination and choice here, with no particular rules to go by. The choice of cleansers is also greater for this skin type – either the wash-off or cream versions will do the job. Moisturize only the areas that need it, and do not forget that your skin is a living organism, and as such it changes. Summer and winter months call for different amounts of product, applied in different places.

SENSITIVE SKIN

Nearly everybody experiences the odd allergic reaction at some point, but truly sensitive skin is quite rare. If you are unlucky enough to have the kind of complexion that flares up frequently, treat it as if it were dry: avoid harsh products that contain alcohol or surfactants (detergents used in certain cleansers and soaps), and choose products that are not highly scented. Beware the 'fragrance-free' label, however, as often this means that yet more chemicals are included to mask an otherwise noticeable scent. Although the concept of natural ingredients is an attractive one, remember that sensitive skin can often react violently to products with live plant extracts. Instead, look for products that are labelled 'hypoallergenic' (but check the contents just in case), especially ones that contain skin soothers such as kaolin, camomile and aloe. These days even make-up is packaged with extensive ingredients lists – check your cosmetics in the same way you check your skincare, and you will minimize unpleasant reactions. Avoid the sun entirely or protect yourself with a high-factor chemical sunscreen such as titanium dioxide.

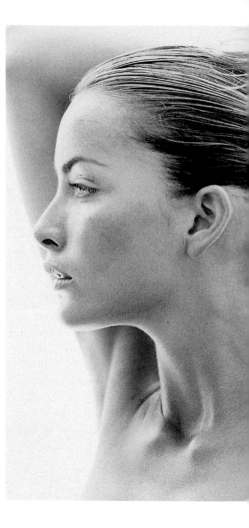

skincare

CLEANSING

Step one in everybody's make-up regime should be thorough cleansing – let's face it, if you were going to spray-paint your car you would first wash off the grimy bits sticking to its surface. While cleansing is at the core of a traditional beauty regime, it is also at the heart of the dermatologist–cosmetologist debate. While old-school dermatologists insist that soap with water is the only way to cleanse the skin thoroughly, most women know from bitter experience that this is a sure way to a dry and itchy face. Although soap is frequently maligned as a surface stripper, many bars contain fats that leave superficial traces, and these can lead to clogged pores and unsightly break-outs. Despite its reputation for harshness, soap is alkaline while the skin itself is acidic – used too frequently, soap can impair the skin's acid mantle (its pH balance) and deplete its defences.

If you are unfortunate enough to look like a walking advertisement for olive oil, the temptation to scrub your skin clean with soapy water can be all-consuming. After all, there is nothing like a good 'rub 'n' suds' routine to leave you feeling fresher. However, if you feel grimy following anything but a

'When your skin changes, as a result of climate, age, stress or other factors, your skincare system needs to be adjusted accordingly. Compare it to when you first join a professional gym. A trained instructor will assess your individual fitness level before determining your personal fitness programme, and as you improve (or maybe get injured) your system needs to be either up- or downgraded. The same idea applies to skincare.'

**Susan Steitzer,
former vice president,
Education, Clinique**

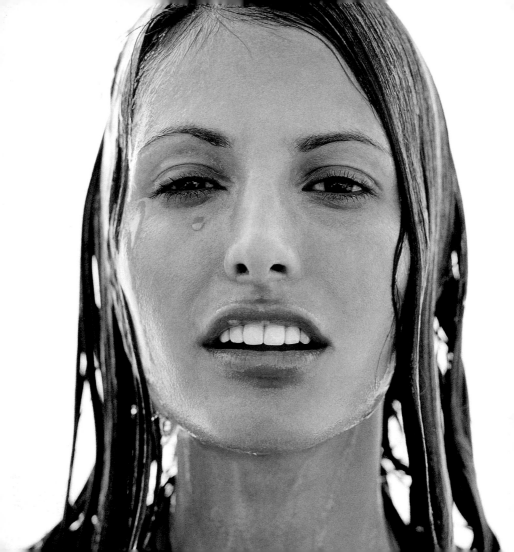

water-based routine, there are now a plethora of wash-off products on the market (everything from bars to foams to liquid cleansers) that are just as satisfying to use, and milder on the complexion. Avoid ingredients such as lanolin, paraffin and added moisturizers, as they block the pores and lead to break-outs; and leave anything containing the extremely drying benzoyl peroxide to the acne-conscious teenager. Remember that although a non-soap cleanser will set you back a little more than the average bar of Lux, your face will not feel like a wrung-out face cloth an hour after you have washed it.

If the driest thing about you is not your sense of humour, you are best treating your face to a milky or cream cleanser. Made

CLEANSING TIPS

1 Wash your hands first. Dirty paws make for dirty faces.

2 Cleanse well around the edges of your face – remember that make-up travels round your jaw line, and after a good night out most hair products end up past your hairline.

3 Change your cleanser with the weather – harsh winds in winter and hot sun in summer can be drying and affect the behaviour of the epidermis.

4 If you have sensitive skin, use a mild cream cleanser. Avoid anything that contains lanolin or fragrance, as these can aggravate the skin and lead to soreness.

5 Do not use the same bottle of cleanser for more than eight to ten weeks. Like everything else, skincare has sell-by dates, and these should be respected if you want to maximize the benefits.

of oil-in-water emulsions, they remove make-up effectively, while still leaving a little moisture on the surface. Oils should be left for the frying pan, or those who suffer from chronic dryness, as although they promise to leave no greasy residue, they are usually rich enough to cleanse an elephant.

TONING

These days toners have definitely gone out of fashion. Modern opinion is that faces do not need toning as skin tone comes from within, and cannot be applied from a bottle. However, the superficial tightening effect of these products, which are generally astringent, is a good preparation for foundation, as it makes any open pores look smaller – albeit temporarily. But be warned: if you use toner too often you could end up suffering from dry, tight skin. In addition, watch out for 'clarifying' mists and lotions – they may glory in modern names, but they still often contain harsh skincare agents such as acids, alcohol and witch hazel. However, if you do not feel properly cleansed unless you make toning a regular part of your beauty regime, make sure that you choose a product that is alcohol free.

MOISTURIZING

To say you do not use moisturizer is tantamount to heresy in the beauty world. However, some people manage to live perfectly happy lives without it. Understanding the natural moisture levels of your own skin is key to finding the right type of moisturizer to suit you. The idea that simply categorizing yourself as 'greasy', 'dry' or 'normal' is the answer to moisturizing seems archaic. Today we all know that a combination of external factors such as changing weather and a hostile environment, and inner factors such as stress and fluctuating hormones, mean your skin has different needs at different times, and that these needs are always individual and specific to you.

The water flow from the dermis to the surface of the skin, and the sebum that forms a barrier on the surface of the skin to delay water evaporation, are what determine your skin's moisture levels. As we age, both the levels of sebum and the levels of water present decrease. Areas that did not need moisturizing before may suddenly feel dry and require a little extra help.

Long gone are the days when moisturizer was nothing but a simple pot of cold cream (although many a dermatologist will tell you that simple cold cream is all your skin requires). Today, thanks to revolutions in skincare technology, creams at both ends of the market contain ingredients that are anti-ageing, anti-pollutant, anti-ultraviolet and antioxidant, to name but a few. No longer the humble potion knocked up in someone's kitchen, today's skincare has huge scientific laboratories and scores of researchers working behind it. We now not only understand the composition and function of human skin, but can also simulate it, making it possible to deliver active ingredients right into its deepest layers. The

Only use a moisturizer where you need it. You cannot hydrate skin properly using topical applications alone – you have to drink plenty of water. Open-pored areas do not like being moisturized. People with combined oily patches and dry patches think that they should moisturize, but I think that they should exfoliate. You cannot stick peeling flakes of skin back down and expect them to attach to the surface.'

Eve Lom, skincare expert

sceptic once sneered at the idea that creams could penetrate so deeply; today the Food and Drug Administration in the USA keeps tight checks on all ingredients, in case something that is strong enough to be classed as a prescription drug is passed off as a simple face cream.

While there is a moisturizer in every texture and for every skin type, they always fall into two main categories: these are humectants and occlusives. The humectant variety draws water up from inside the dermis to hydrate the superficial layers, or attracts it from the surrounding atmosphere. Occlusives (better for drier skins) create an oily film on the surface of your complexion, and this seals moisture in and prevents evaporation. There are oil-free water emulsions for oily skins (look for products labelled non-comedogenic as these help prevent unsightly break-outs) and water-in-oil formulations for drier skins. Whatever your skin type, a good tip is to make sure that your face is slightly damp before you apply moisturizer – this will make it go further, and remove the temptation to slap on great globules of unnecessary product.

EYES

The eyes are windows to the soul and give a clear insight into your beauty regimen. The area round the eyes is the first to show fine lines and wrinkles, so the temptation to overdo eye cream is enormous. But less is more when it comes to eye care. One Harley Street plastic surgeon insists that most of the patients who come to him wanting blepharoplasty

'The skin around the eyes does not contain open pores. It has very little adipose tissue, and should therefore be protected. Use a cream thick enough to stand the heat and cold, but make sure it is matt, not oily.'

Eve Lom, skincare expert

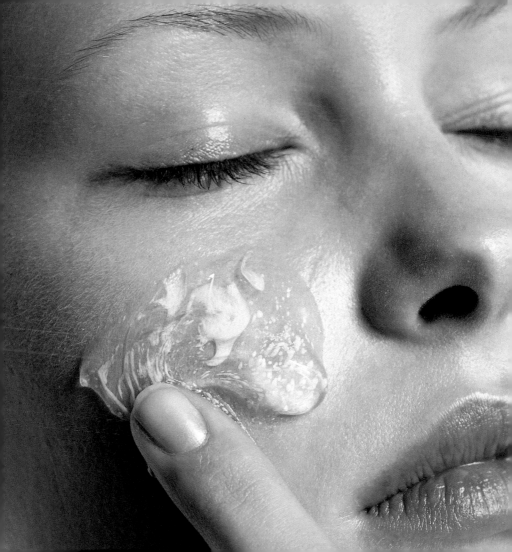

(eye-job) operations have created their under-eye bags by using so much eye gel that it has not been fully absorbed. Rather than risk accumulating eye gel in your sockets, stick with a light cream product and use it sparingly, just dotted around the orbital bone.

While dark circles are often genetic, they can also be the result of poor circulation, alcohol or toxins. Because the skin is so fine underneath the eye, the bluish tint of the underlying blood vessels can sometimes be seen. While companies such as Chanel and Estée Lauder have products to fight dark circles, the most effective strategy is to conceal them. Do not dismiss wet tea bags and cucumber slices as old wives' tales if you suffer from baggy eyes. They act like a poultice to draw out excess fluids and work wonders the morning after the night before.

NECK

The neck and décolletage are two of the sexiest parts of the body when we are young, and two of the least attractive as we get older. Make sure you take care of your neck and chest area with one of the excellent anti-ageing neck creams on the market (Clarins, Estée Lauder and Guerlain all make good ones). Do not wait until it is just too late.

LIPS

If women were allowed to use only one item of make-up, most of us would choose lipstick. As a result, it is slightly surprising that when it comes to taking care of our kissers, most of us are guilty of neglect. Remember that the lips do not have a strong lipid barrier, so they dry out quickly, and the habit of constant licking makes this dehydration worse. The lips have no sebaceous glands either, which makes them almost totally reliant on external moisturizer to keep them in peak condition. The best thing you can do to achieve a perfect pair of pouters is treat them to a daily ritual: first exfoliate (brush them very gently with a toothbrush if you do not want to splash out on a special cream), then hydrate with a protective balm. Remember that smoking and exposure to harmful ultraviolet rays cause ugly vertical lines to appear around the mouth, so invest in a product with UV protection and never leave home without it and, ideally, try to stop smoking.

HANDS

Forget the face-lift: if you haven't taken care of your hands they will be a sure giveaway of your age. Prone to liver spots, lines, wrinkles and general dryness, hands should always be protected from the sun. If you don't want to invest in a separate hand cream, rub your hands together after applying your facial moisturizer (make sure it contains UV protection). On a more mundane level, always wear rubber gloves when you are washing up – a far from glamorous look, this precaution will reap dividends in the long term.

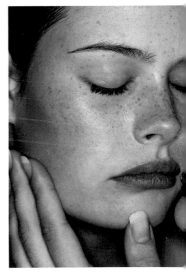

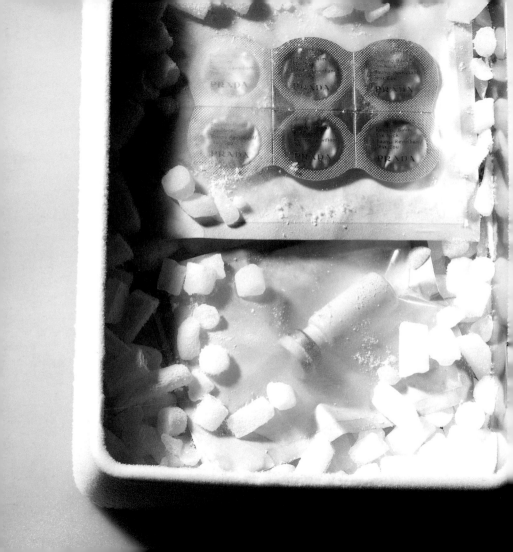

anti-ageing

'With serious signs of ageing such as wrinkles and skin discoloration being such an important focus for the ageing baby-boomer (and therefore the cosmetics industry), the trend for scientifically based products is in great demand. Women are now more aware of the science behind the products, and are demanding more serious, factual explanations about how the products work, and the results that can be expected.'

Shirley Weinstein, senior vice president,
Global Product Development, Clinique

Why should you grow old noticeably? Thanks to a revolution in skincare technology, there is no reason why you should not look as young as you feel for as long as you want to. I am not suggesting that a middle-aged woman should have (or even want) the face of a teenager (in today's world being beautiful does not have to mean being young), merely that she should not have to resign herself to the signs of premature skin ageing. Our genes are partly responsible for how our skin ages over the years (that is, intrinsic ageing), but research is showing more and more clearly that to a large extent, skin ageing is determined by our lifestyle and our environment (that is, extrinsic ageing).

'Most of us live in an environment that overwhelms the skin's own ability to protect itself,' says Dr Daniel Maes, president of Research and Development for Estée Lauder. Smoking, drinking caffeine and alcohol, being exposed to everyday pollution and harmful UV rays, and even not getting enough sleep all have detrimental effects on our faces. Free radicals attack our skin at a cellular level, the collagen and elastin fibres are broken down, and the DNA of the cells is damaged, meaning fewer healthy cells eventually reach the surface.

So what are the signs of ageing skin? The first giveaways are fine lines and wrinkles developing around the eyes (the muscles here are the most mobile in the face and they also take the brunt of all our emotions), followed by a slack, greyish lustre, pigmentation marks, flakiness and a loss of tissue softness. At the menopause women suffer from a sharp fall in epidermal oil and moisture production, which brings about a rapid decline in skin condition – this is one of the reasons that women appear to age faster than men. According to the Research and Development department at La Prairie skincare: 'The older we get, the more cell-renewal time slows down, from about 28 days to about 40 days. Fewer renewed cells reach the surface in older skin, and dead cells at the surface clog together so that plumpness and firmness are depleted.'

Luckily all is not lost, so before you trade in your face creams for a Balaclava, rest assured that science is on your side. Today beauty companies are using DNA technology to slow down the ageing process of the skin by encouraging cells to split and renew, and even fight the harmful effects of the sun at a cellular level. 'We can foresee that in the distant future we may not need any sunscreens to provide us with UV protection, as the increased defence capacity of the skin cells will allow the skin to remain protected. The discovery of heat-shock proteins in the skin cells, which provide protection against UV damage, is a major step forward. It means we are now developing technologies that will allow a more natural way for the cells to repair themselves,' says Dr Maes.

If the future of skincare seems almost space age, the present is not that far behind. We are already able to grow whole sheets of human skin under laboratory conditions, and have made substantial technological breakthroughs that are scientifically proven to help reverse the effects of premature ageing.

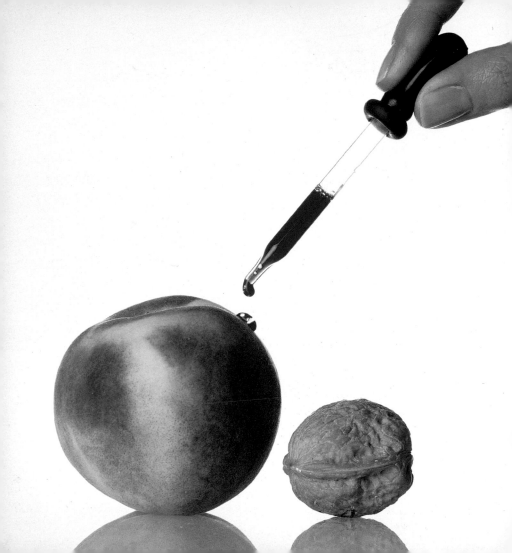

miracles in a jar

Science has revolutionized skincare, and thanks to many years of research and development we really are now able to turn back the clock in the constant battle against ageing. Here are some of the most striking weapons in our armoury:

ALPHA-HYDROXY ACIDS (AHAS)

Hated by some but loved by many, these were one among the most significant discoveries in the fight against ageing during the twentieth century. AHAs include glycolic, lactic, malic, tartaric and citric acids, all naturally found in fruit and milk. Exfoliant and mildly abrasive, they dissolve the intercellular glue that sticks dead cells to the surface of the skin, and encourage desquamation (the natural shedding of the cells). Healthy new cells thus reach the surface quicker. At best this gives you a more youthful appearance, and improves the texture and colour of your skin. It also makes your skin appear plumper, because AHAs boost the moisture retention of the skin. However, they do not have a cumulative effect, so this added moisture is only present while you are using the creams. On the downside, many people have developed allergic reactions to AHAs. They are prone to sensitize the skin, and if you are using them you must be protected by a sunscreen at all times.

BETA HYDROXY ACIDS

These are also exfoliant, but slightly less irritant than AHAs. Often used to treat acne (BHAs such as salicylic acid remove oil from pores), they help reduce fine lines and fade pigmentation marks. As with AHAs, they can cause the skin to be photosensitive, so sunscreens must always be worn in tandem with them.

RETINOIDS

Hailed as a miracle cure for acne, a retinoid is an anti-ageing ingredient derived from Vitamin A. Retinoids come in different forms (such as Renova, Retinova, Retin-A and retinol), and unclog pores, allowing sebum to travel freely to the surface. Users swear they improve skin texture and the appearance of surface lines and wrinkles, although the Advertising Standards Authority in the UK has recently questioned this claim. Downsides are that these creams can sting on application and may leave the skin red and flaky for several weeks afterwards. Vitamin A impairs wound healing, so avoid aggressive treatments such as waxing while using these creams. Photosensitivity is possible, so remember to always wear sunscreen.

VITAMIN C

A powerful antioxidant, vitamin C boosts the production of collagen in the skin. This, in turn, slows down the development of wrinkles and helps repair sun damage. Vitamin C is now used in various skincare products and is a proven way of slowing down the clock.

NATURAL PLANT INGREDIENTS

While the appliance of science has catapulted the beauty industry into the futuristic world of discovery that it now proudly inhabits, some of the most potent ingredients are still sourced from the bounty of mother nature. As a result, Liz Earle, botanical beauty expert, has formulated her entire Naturally Active Skincare range around some of these natural beauty enhancers.

ECHINACEA Not just a popular remedy for the common cold, echinacea is also known for its skin-strengthening properties. 'It promotes skin regeneration and encourages the production of fibroplasts, which form the supporting structure of the skin,' says Liz.

ALOE VERA A natural ingredient of near-mythical status, aloe vera is used across the world for both its healing and its soothing properties.

ARGAN OIL Organically extracted from a Moroccan tree of the same name, this is rich in vitamin E, an antioxidant that helps to combat skin ageing.

SKINCARE JARGON

ANTIOXIDANTS These form the body's best defence system against free-radical damage, which leads to premature ageing. Vitamins E and C and betacarotene are all used in face creams, but they should also be incorporated into your diet on a regular basis.

LIPIDS These are not active ingredients but a delivery system. They help the skin to absorb active ingredients.

CERAMIDES These are used in moisturizers because they are wonderful water-binding agents. They are present in healthy skin, but dry and dehydrated complexions are often deficient in them.

KERATIN This is a protein found naturally in skin and hair. It is often used as a strengthener in shampoos and other hair-care products.

COLLAGEN AND ELASTIN These are the fibres that plump up skin and give it elasticity. The production of both collagen and elastin lessens with age, causing skin to become slack and lose its youthful appearance. Applied topically, collagen and elastin lend a superficial firmness to the skin because they are very efficient at absorbing water.

HUMECTANTS These attract moisture from the surrounding atmosphere, or the dermis to the epidermis. Glycerol and sorbitol are both effective humectants in the treatment of dry skin.

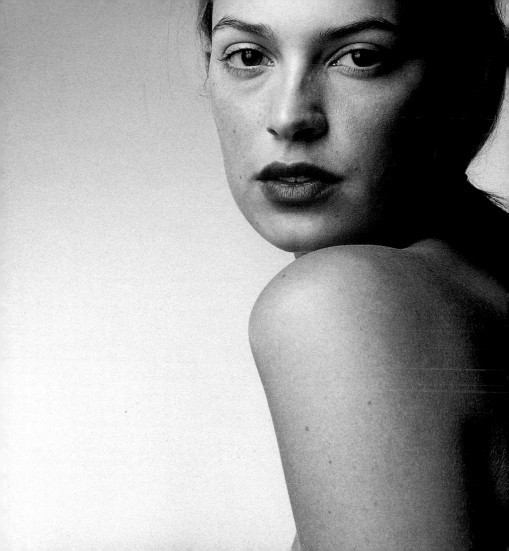

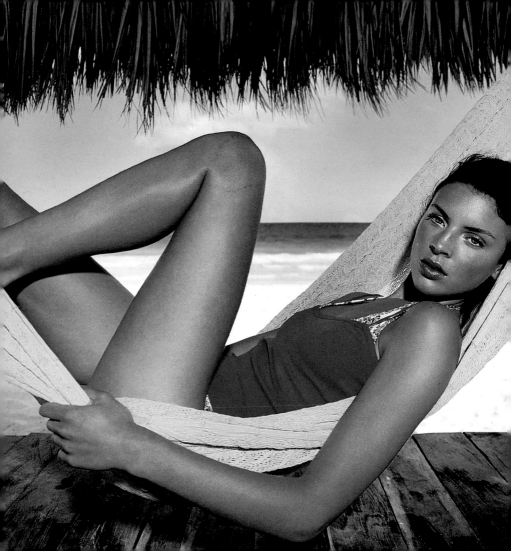

sun skin

Undoubtedly, a spot of sunbathing gives you a glowing tan that can make you look and feel good, but remember that you are under attack from heat and ultraviolet rays. Sunlight breaks down collagen and elastin fibres and damages the skin cells (UVA rays lead to ageing, UVB to burning), and while olive skin is less at risk from damage, it still requires a sunscreen. As Dr David Orentreich, Clinique's guiding dermatologist says: 'The single worst thing you can do to your skin is overexpose it to the sun. Ninety per cent of the damage seen on the skin in the form of ageing (lines, wrinkles, discoloration) is due to sun exposure.'

LIFE'S A BEACH

While most of us are well acquainted with the dangers of the sun, we are less aware of the dangers of the water. A dip in the ocean may be an instant refresher but if you're not careful it can add to the frying factor on the beach:

1 Never dry off naturally after a swim. Water droplets act as mini magnifying glasses and intensify the strength of the sun's rays.

2 Always take a shower immediately after a swim. Remember that sea water contains salt and pool water contains chemicals, both of which are very drying for the skin.

3 Protect your hair. Daily dips in salt water and chlorine will wreak havoc on your locks, so invest in a hair product that contains a protective layer of silicone, as well as UV protection. This will act as a sealant, to keep colour and condition in, and salt and chemicals out.

4 Increase your sun protection factor (SPF). Whether you're water-skiing or simply relaxing on a boat, the reflection of the sun's glare is a serious threat to your skin. Use a waterproof sunscreen and reapply it regularly, particularly after swimming.

5 Always sit in the shade. Wear sunglasses with UV protection whenever you are on or near the water to avoid damage to your eyes from the reflected glare. Attach your sunglasses with a cord around your neck so that you won't lose them if you fall in.

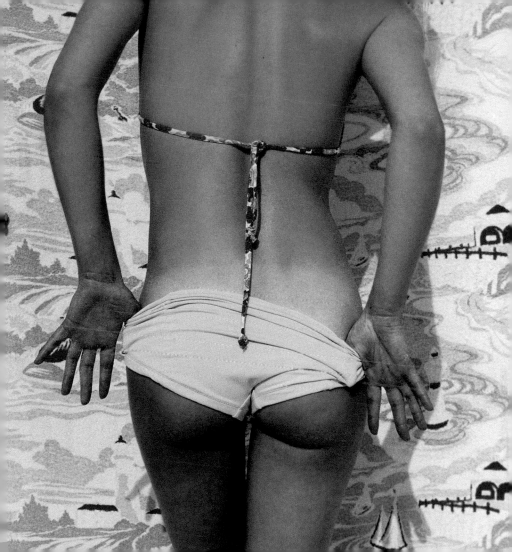

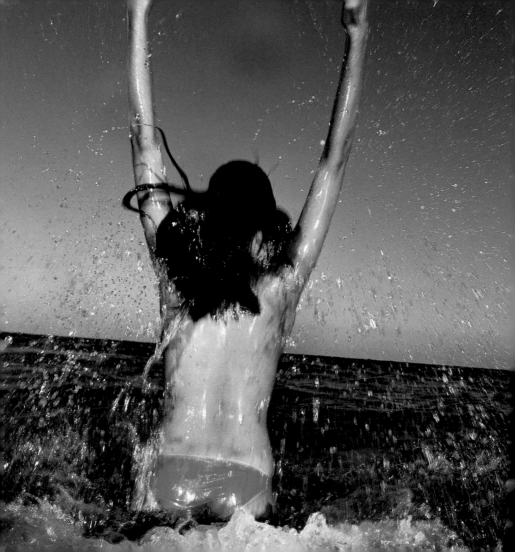

SAFE SUN TIPS

1 Always wear a moisturizer with a sun protection factor (SPF), even on a cloudy day.

2 Apply your sunscreen 15 minutes before hitting the sun to give it time to be absorbed.

3 Make sure your sunscreen is broad spectrum and contains both UVA and UVB protection. Look for chemical ingredients such as avobenzone, which absorbs and deactivates rays, or physical ingredients such as titanium dioxide, which blocks the rays and bounces them away from the skin, so that they are no longer dangerous. (Don't worry – today's products have been refined, so they won't leave you looking like a snowman.)

4 Reapply your sunscreen regularly, not just after swimming. Remember that even a waterproof lotion can be rubbed off by your towel.

5 Know your SPFs. Everybody can stay out in the sun for an average of five to ten minutes without burning; the number on the bottle indicates how much you can multiply this by when protected by the sunscreen. Remember that SPFs are not cumulative – rubbing in a factor 10 on top of a factor 20 does not give you SPF 30.

6 Wear a higher SPF on your face than on your body, as this is the area you will most want to protect from ageing.

7 Have moles checked regularly, particularly any that appear after exposure to the sun.

8 Always wear sunglasses with UV-filtered lenses to protect your eyes from the glare of the sun.

FAKING IT

You can now glory in all the glamour of a month-in-the-Med tan without any of the subsequent dangers caused by roasting yourself in the sun. Today's fake tans are more realistic than ever before – they are non-streak, non-smelly and they fade evenly. For the best results, follow these application tips:

1 First, exfoliate well to make sure you have a smooth body surface. (A salon treatment will deal with those hard-to-reach places.) If you prefer to do it yourself, a body mitt is a good alternative to a body scrub, but should never be used on the face. Alternatively, there are umpteen exfoliating creams and foams on the market, all of which smell delicious and add a little luxury to the treatment. For a totally smooth canvas, exfoliate at least twice before applying your fake tan.

2 Make sure your skin is squeaky clean and truly dry to prevent the tan trickling down your legs and on to the bathroom floor.

3 Choose the correct colour and texture for you. There are now gels, sprays, mousses and lotions to suit every skin type and colour. Be sure to rub the tan in evenly, and to guarantee a non-streak finish, wait ten minutes before getting dressed.

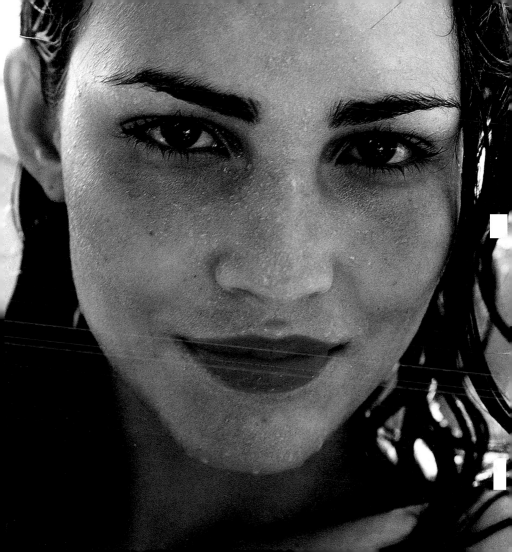

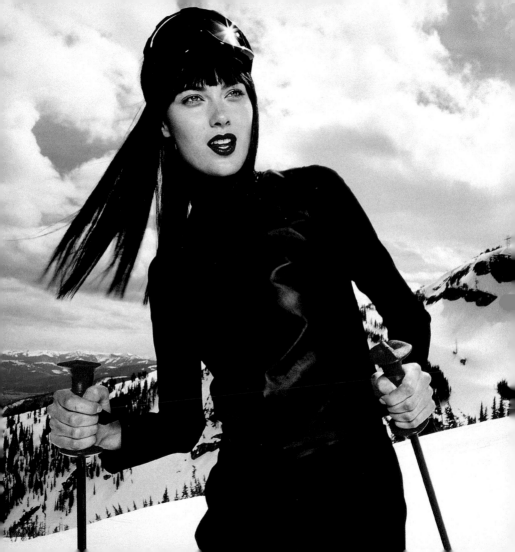

4 Pay particular attention to bony places – knees, elbows and noses are sure telltale areas if you do not rub the product in properly. Mix your tan with a moisturizer before applying it to your face – this will tone it down and help give an even application.

5 Wash your hands when you have finished to avoid being left with orange palms.

SKI SKIN

There are few things in life more exhilarating than whizzing down the ski slopes to earn some après-ski fun and relaxation. But while most of your body is well covered for the majority of the time, your face and hands are often exposed to the sun's powerful rays, which are made even stronger than in normal conditions because they are reflected off the snow. Remember that sun protection is just as crucial on the slopes as it is on the beach, so next time you slip into your ski suit, remember to follow a few simple guidelines. If you're going to get piste, don't let the gluhwein go to your head.

1 Remember that the snow acts like a mirror – it reflects the sun's rays, making them far more powerful and far more dangerous, even if it feels cold. Always use a total sunblock, and do not be persuaded otherwise by a whistling wind or low cloud cover. Maximum protection is vital at all times.

2 Do not forget your extremities: lips and ears tend to burn more on the slopes because they are easily forgotten. Physical barriers such as titanium dioxide are especially good for lips. Remember to coat your nose, forehead and neck with total sunblock.

3 Always wear glasses or goggles with good protective lenses. These are worth the expense because reflected UV rays are extremely harmful to the eyes, and in some cases cause snow blindness.

4 Wear a hat – most of your body heat is lost through your head – or, if you prefer not to, protect your hair with a UV hair product. Do not forget that your hair is just as likely to be damaged by the sun on the piste as on the beach.

JET LAG SKIN

'I fly constantly and try to drink as much water as I can throughout the flight. I apply Sundãri's Neem Cream regularly when I fly. Neem is an indigenous ingredient from the Indian Himalayas and has many healing properties. It is also a natural antiseptic and deeply hydrating,' says supermodel Christy Turlington.

Flying can wreak havoc on the skin. The combination of cabin pressure and dehydration cause skin to look grey and old. Take a few precautions before you hit the tarmac:

1 Make sure you drink plenty of water (not alcohol) on the flight. Cabin air is drier than the Sahara Desert, so keep drinking water throughout. Avoid caffeine, too, as it is dehydrating.

2 Do not wear make-up. It is guaranteed to look awful by the time you land, not to mention making your skin feel tight during the flight. Use a moisturizer such as Prescriptives Flight Cream to ensure your skin retains its water levels until you land.

3 Walk up and down the aisle, if at all feasible, and do leg exercises (rotate ankles up and down, and in alternate directions) every half hour to avoid water retention and sluggish circulation.

4 Prevent static hair with a product such as Kiehl's Silk Groom. Taking a satin pillowcase with you will also help, as airline pillows create chaos with your hair.

5 Take on board an aromatherapy kit specifically designed for flying. Daniele Ryman and Aromatherapeutics make great ones that will keep you awake or help you sleep, as well as protect you from the many germs that are rife in recirculated cabin air.

6 Remember that getting over a flight can be more stressful than getting on one. The Hale Clinic offers renowned light-therapy treatments to jet lag sufferers, which are worth the investment.

problem skin

However flawless our natural complexion, everybody suffers from problem skin at some time or another. Stress, an aggressive environment and hormonal fluctuations can all contribute to distressing break-outs. But you don't have to suffer in silence:

• Do not get depressed – easier said than done, but angst may lead to more spots.

• Remember that not suffering from acne as a teenager does not make you immune for life: many women who were blemish free in their youth suffer in their twenties. This can mean a decade of misery, but the acne generally disappears during their thirties.

• Avoid food with high levels of saturated fat. Treat deep-fried foods as public enemy number one, and do not indulge in too many dairy products, which can contribute to blocked pores and the onset of pimples.

• Drink plenty of filtered water, and eat as many portions of fresh fruit and vegetables as you can manage (five a day is the recommended daily amount). Steaming your vegetables is the best way to maintain their valuable mineral and vitamin content if you do not want to eat them raw.

• Tie your hair back at night to prevent grease travelling down your forehead, and wash your hair regularly. Avoid using too many hair products, as they can aggravate the skin and lead to break-outs.

• Steer clear of any harsh skincare products – they will only exacerbate the problem.

• Resist temptation – make it a cast-iron rule never to pick your spots, as you will inflame the tissue around the blemish and cause infection to spread.

• If problem skin persists, consult a dermatologist. It may be that over-the-counter remedies are doing nothing for you and you should try a Retin-A cream (prescription only), instead. Retin-A can work miracles with acne, but it is also very strong and does have side effects. As a result, make sure that your dermatologist tells you about any contraindications before you start a course.

• Exercise regularly – this is the best way to get your whole system working to its full potential, and also helps the body to eliminate waste.

• Sleep well – there's nothing quite like eight hours of peaceful slumber to help your skin to heal itself, and promote a clear and refined complexion.

diet

When all is said and done, make-up and topical skincare applications only add a superficial varnish to the full picture. Remember that inner health makes for outer beauty, and if you want the outside to look its best you have to nourish the inside. So the next time you feel pangs of hunger, it is worth reminding yourself that you really are what you eat and choose sensibly.

RED WINE taken in moderation has a marvellous effect on your health. The grapes used to produce the wine contain powerful and vitalizing antioxidants.

GREEN TEA is not just popular as an accompaniment to sushi. It boosts the immune system, and contains ingredients that help fight cancer as well as combat free radicals.

STRAWBERRIES are deliciously rich in vitamin C. They help the body absorb iron from other foods in the diet, and act as a general cleanser.

GARLIC will do more for your health than for your social life. It contains minerals that increase your energy levels, and a host of antioxidants to combat ageing.

ECHINACEA has long been popular in the USA to ward off colds and flu, and is widely gaining recognition as an anti-ageing remedy. In its raw state it is a herb with antibiotic properties.

BANANAS contain a high concentration of potassium and natural sugar. This sugar is quickly absorbed and raises energy levels for far longer than the refined sugars in chocolate do, making bananas a popular snack for athletes.

LIVE YOGURT (with acidophilus) helps maintain the natural bacteria present in the gut, so it is particularly beneficial to eat it if you are taking antibiotics (which tend to destroy the bacteria). It also protects you from bowel infections and can be used to treat thrush.

CRANBERRIES AND CRANBERRY JUICE are natural diuretics, flush the system, and are often used to combat cystitis.

BEETROOT is an effective cleanser. When it is included in a healthy diet it helps to flush toxins from the blood and kidneys.

CELERY is amazingly low in calories (just four a stick). Munching on this healthy snack will benefit your figure and your complexion.

GREEN CABBAGE and spring greens are both high in iron. They are a fantastic source of other minerals and nutrients (particularly if you do not eat red meat) and aid in children's healthy development.

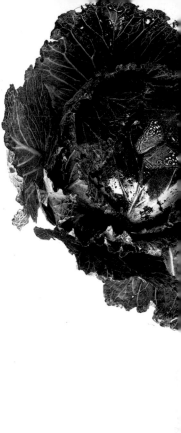

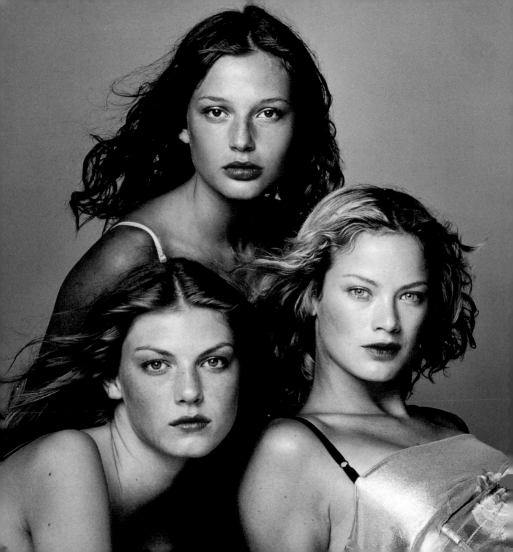

face shapes

'I love strong features on a woman and I find them a powerful element of beauty.'

Bobbi Brown, make-up guru

Despite an obsession with the ins and outs of skincare, most women slap on make-up with total disregard for their bone structure. We spend months improving our complexions, and then wreck the final look because we just do not understand our faces well enough.

Think of applying make-up as a final couture dress fitting – to make the silk lie smoothly you have to follow the pattern. So next time you sit down with powder and paint, close your eyes and tap gently around your features. These are the foundations upon which you will always work – they define your ultimate possibilities as well as your limits. Instead of wishing for somebody else's face (and yes, we have all done it), take note of your strong or unusual features. Remember that these are what make you beautiful – they differentiate you from the crowd, and compose the badge of your individuality.

CELEBRITIES WITH DISTINCTIVE FEATURES

MADONNA Heart-shaped face, and gap between the teeth.
SARAH JESSICA PARKER Prominent nose and jaw line.
PALOMA PICASSO Hooded eyes and big nose.
CALISTA FLOCKHART Wide mouth.
MINNIE DRIVER Prominent jaw.
JEMIMA KHAN Roman nose.
CHLOË SEVIGNY Distinctive nose and generally quirky features.

Accept your prominent nose or strong jaw line and resolve to accentuate rather than hide it. Today, beauty is not the exclusive domain of the lucky few with regular features. Whatever your face shape, beauty is at your fingertips – acquire a detailed understanding of who you are, and use this knowledge to your advantage.

DIFFERENT FACE SHAPES

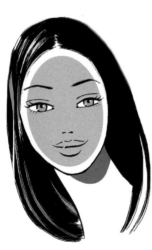

THE OVAL FACE Historically considered the most beautiful, in this face shape the features are evenly spaced and balanced and render make-up application easy. Emmanuelle Béart, Penélope Cruz

THE ROUND FACE (OR 'BUTTON') Usually combined with a small nose, this face shape can (often misleadingly) give the immediate impression of chubbiness. Cameron Diaz, Emma Bunton, Drew Barrymore

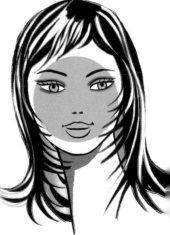

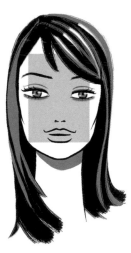

THE LONG FACE (OR 'HORSE') Defined by a powerful jaw, the long face gives the owner an appearance of strength, and sometimes hardness. Make-up is used best as a softener. Jerry Hall, Kylie Minogue, Jennifer Aniston

THE SQUARE FACE The jaw, when seen from the side, is almost at right angles to the jaw bone. Accentuating the upper third of the face gives a soft, doe-eyed look. Isabella Rossellini, Audrey Hepburn

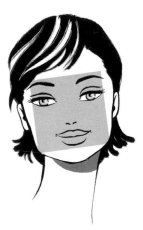

THE HEART-SHAPED FACE Defined by wide cheekbones and a pointy chin, the heart-shaped face gives an impression of girlie femininity. Minnie Driver, Helena Bonham Carter

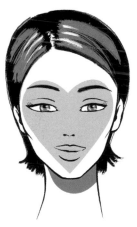

tricks of the trade

'Make-up isn't about rules, it's about options,' says Bobbi Brown, and of course there are times when you wish to tone down your strongest features. After all, if you want to look great, you certainly need to feel it. The art of optical illusion has always played a vital role in the history of make-up. From its earliest days as tribal war paint, right up to its most sophisticated application today, it has been used to disguise and enhance. For those who wish to change their look (with no intention of braving a surgeon's knife), shading and highlighting are the most effective ways to alter your features. Celebrity make-up artist Ruby Hammer of Ruby & Millie make-up has a few trade secrets to help you make the most (or least) of your features:

SLIM A WIDE NOSE

Make-up is just about the interplay of light and dark. Light colours push areas out; dark colours force them to recede. The best way to slim down a podgy nose is by doing some clever highlighting and shading. Use a light-coloured highlighter, not a shimmery one. MAC's taupe shadow is a good shader, and Ruby & Millie make 'face enhancers' (a compact containing a highlighter and a shader) in three colours. Photographers also use light to bring out certain features and disguise others, but real life isn't like that. Be very light-handed in your application and only use this method at night. If you hit the beach with a shaded nose, a friend may offer to rub it for you, mistakenly thinking it's dirty.

1 When you apply your highlighter and shader, make sure that you put them on over your foundation.

2 Using a soft-haired brush – I prefer synthetic ones since they're less hairy – apply a highlighter down the centre of the nose (top).

3 Contour it with a darker colour on either side (bottom).

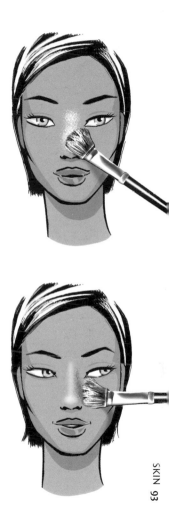

CREATE A FULL MOUTH

This is far more achievable for daily life.

1 Instead of outlining with lip pencil first, go for a plumping product (there are plenty on the market, but BeneFit's Lip Plump is a good one) to fill in the lines.

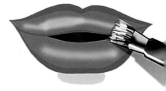

2 As far as colour goes, anything that is neither matt nor flat will look more lush, which is why glosses are so popular. Remember that your lips are mobile (only pouting models caught in a single photographic image are static), so the mouth you create will have to withstand activities such as talking, eating and drinking.

3 Next use a lip primer and, with a lip brush, apply a colour that's a little creamy all over the natural lip line, and slightly over the edges. Blot, and reapply colour.

4 Then use a lip pencil to boost the upper-lip shape. I don't like using more liner than this because in real life you are seen from 360°, and a total lip line looks false.

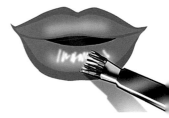

5 Top up the mouth with a little extra gloss on the centre of the lower lip, and in the Cupid's bow of the upper lip.

MINIMIZE THE FOREHEAD

This is partly down to make-up, and partly down to hairstyle.

1 To disguise a very prominent brow, it's important that you resist the temptation to scrape your hair back off your face.

2 Cutting in a few layers down the sides of the face detracts attention from it.

3 Play up two other strong features – the eyes and the lips to balance things out.

4 Apply a sparing amount of shadow along the hairline to make it recede (right). But don't do this in hot weather, or when you are likely to get sweaty – after all, you don't want a smudge running down your nose.

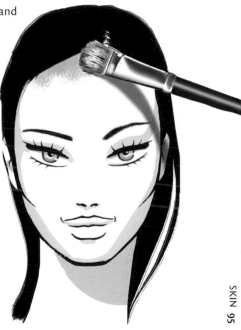

OPEN HOODED EYES

Most people try to reverse hooded eyes by sweeping eyeshadow up and outwards. However, I find that this draws more attention to any folds of skin. Try the following tips instead.

1 Coat the entire lid with a neutral wash of colour – a mushroomy shade works well – and then highlight with a paler colour on the brow bone (top).

2 Next take a darker, defining colour, and concentrate it close to the eyelashes (bottom). This will bring out the eyes and diminish the hooded look. Remember that eyes become increasingly hooded with age, and skin tone becomes crepey, too. Coloured shadow will crack and draw attention to wrinkles.

3 Finally, apply lots of mascara on upper lashes, and a little colour under the lower ones to balance out the look.

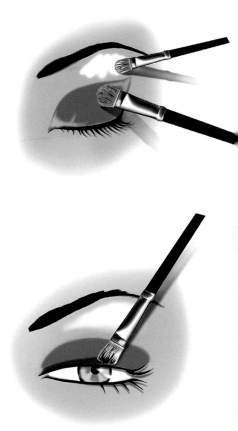

HIDE A RECEDING CHIN

1 Use your normal base colour, and then a shimmery highlighter, dotted on your chin, nose, forehead and the tops of your cheeks (right). The shimmer catches the light and pushes your features forward, giving your face, and chin, a lift.

SHADING AND TONING TIPS

1 Make sure you have a good contouring brush for powder highlighters and shading products. Powder products are best applied on top of your foundation.

2 Invest in cream or liquid highlighters or shaders. These are simple to apply with the fingertips, and wipe off easily if you make a mistake.

3 Do not be put off by the 'zebra' effect of a liquid shadow/highlighter. Apply foundation on top of this.

4 Practise in daylight so you can see what you are doing. Really feel the contours of your face before you start.

5 For a natural evening look, shade and tone by electric light.

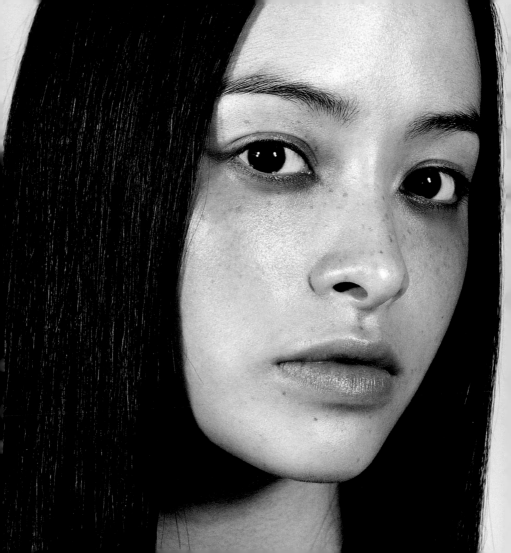

skin tone

'I much prefer people who are noticed for their daring use of colour to people whose make-up choices are so boring that they don't get noticed at all.'

Kevyn Aucoin, make-up artist

With cultural diversity and interracial partnerships reshaping our vision of the ideal, every hair and skin colour makes an equal mark on the beauty map. Ever since Naomi Campbell first graced the cover of *Vogue*, black models such as Veronica Webb and Alek Wek have become increasingly successful, while Asian beauties are paid fortunes for advertising campaigns and glossy magazine shoots (think Devon Aoki and Lucy Liu).

In the modern world, the idea of make-up and skincare aimed specifically at black or Asian skins seems out of date: the plethora of colours and textures offered by companies at both ends of the spectrum covers every individual's needs. Besides, this type of categorizing is exclusive – the opposite of what today's inclusive beauty vision is about.

The same type of liberation applies to hair colour, symbolized by the rising popularity of red, formerly a colour most of us wished to avoid. Today's women cannot go red fast enough. Julia Roberts (auburn), Nicole Kidman (strawberry blonde) and Karen Elson (Titian) have all been powerful ambassadors for the redhead. Thanks to Versace and other trumpeters of colour, fashion and beauty have embraced the full spectrum of possibilities. Clashing colours are no longer a fashion faux pas; a bold statement is something to be strived for, not avoided.

Even foundation (once split simplistically into 'pink-' or 'yellow-toned') has broken free of its shackles. Thanks to technological advances, we can now find shades and textures to mimic our natural skin tone, whether it be midwinter or holiday suntan. According to international make-up guru François Nars, 'Women are taking care of their skin today. You have to adapt to modernity and change. Looking great is not about a lot of make-up, or no make-up, it is about the right make-up, and translucent skin.'

MAKE-UP APPLICATION TIPS

1 To make sure you select the right colour foundation, choose three shades that you think are about right and streak each one over your face and under your jaw line. Only one will completely disappear on your skin and that is the colour you should buy.

2 Ignore out-of-date taboos – when it comes to colour, anything goes. If you want a natural look, stick to shades traditionally associated with your skin tone (warm tones for yellow-based skins and cooler ones for pink skins), but if you really want to make an entrance, chose the opposite extreme. Redheads, for example, will make a far bolder statement in a cool aqua eyeshadow or a piercing pink lipstick than in an earthy brown.

3 Hair is a slightly more complex equation, as your skin tone will always limit your results. Blonde hair against a very olive skin can leave you looking nauseous, while raven locks on an English rose will look more gothic than alluring.

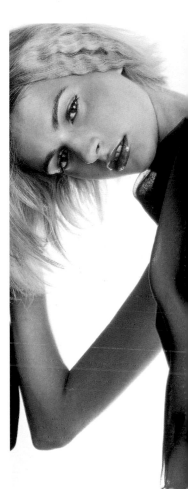

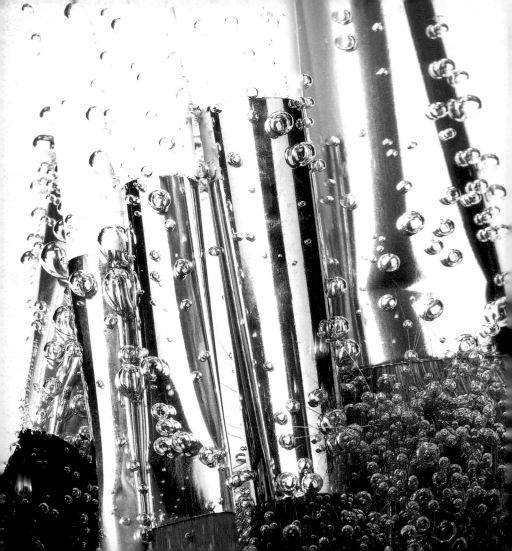

2 tools of the trade

'The right tools make an enormous difference in make-up application. Foundation can be applied more evenly, lip and eye colour can be drawn more efficiently. And it doesn't have to cost a fortune.'

Kevyn Aucoin, make-up artist

Thanks to modern technology, we can all rest assured that our eyeshadow will not flake, our mascara will not clog and our lipstick will not budge. However, what counts is not just what you wear but the way that you wear it, and any girl worth her Chantecaille foundation knows that without exactly the right sponge between her fingers, the result will never be as good as it could be. So refined are colours and textures these days that there is no reason why, given a few handy hints, the canny customer should not always look as if she is going to the Oscars. If we get it wrong, it is usually not our make-up that is at fault, but rather that we have used the wrong kit to apply it. So remember that when it comes to poor make-up application, a bad workman really will be right to blame her tools.

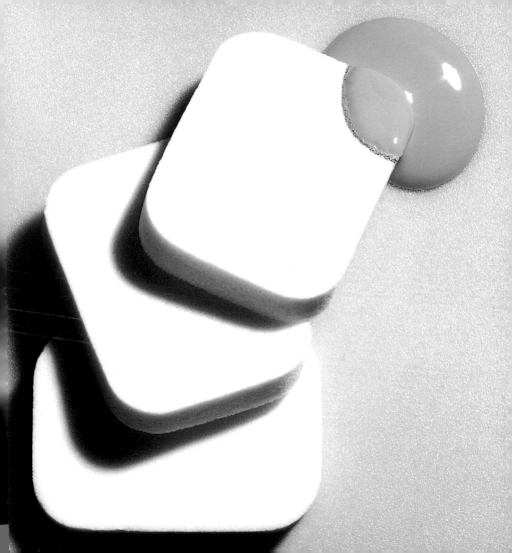

the full monty
(A MAKE-UP ARTIST'S TOOL KIT)

FOUNDATION SPONGES

These are brilliant for building up coverage slowly in layers. For liquid and cream foundations, use a wedge to give you control and help spread it evenly. Avoid natural sponges – use even-textured synthetic ones (make sure they are latex-free), which are soft and malleable.

POWDER BRUSH

This is the time to go 'Hollywood movie'. Invest in the biggest, softest, fluffiest version you can find. Shu Uemura, Ruby & Millie and MAC make wonderful powder brushes. The more generous the head, the more the powder will be diffused – big is definitely beautiful here. Great for applying bronzer, as it gives even coverage all over the face, this tool should not be substituted for a blusher brush, as for that you need a thinner, more angled head to get a clean result.

CONCEALER BRUSH

Definitely go synthetic here. Sable brushes tend to become blocked with cream, whereas a synthetic brush glides smoothly through the product, picking up just enough to distribute evenly. Generally, to help you make the right choice between natural and synthetic brushes for particular tasks, always imagine the texture of the product they will be moving through.

EYESHADOW BRUSH

For the really indulgent, three eyeshadow brushes will take you wherever you want to go in style. A tiny brush allows you to go right up to the eyelash line for fine precision work (when you want to draw a single line, or accentuate the crease in your eyelid). A medium one will pick up a lot of colour and wash it over the lid in a couple of moves, and a big diffuser brush will let you really blend, blend, blend. Resist the temptation to dip this brush into vibrant shadows – save it for applying the neutral base colours that are the staple undercoat for any look.

ANGLED EYEBROW BRUSH

This will be the hardest brush in your collection. Great for giving control to wild eyebrows, it adds a final touch of grooming to a finished look. Brushed upwards, brows look striking in photographs. Origins make a fabulous eyebrow brush, in a dark green lacquer.

LIP BRUSHES

That so many women apply lipstick without a lip brush is shocking – the results are so vastly improved when you use one. Ideally, invest in two lip brushes – the first to do the donkey work, and a second, small retractable one to keep in your handbag. Whether you choose a square-edged brush or a tapered one is up to you: a square-edged one gives more control on line work, while a tapered one lets you get right into the corners. A natural bristle is better here, so if you are going to splash out on a sable brush, this is the time to do it.

EYELASH COMB

Tweezerman and Ruby & Millie produce the best eyelash combs. They have a wonderful section for separating the lashes on one end and a brush to temper the lashes with (once the mascara has dried) on the other.

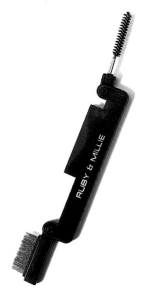

EYEBROW STENCILS

These make shaping the eyebrow far easier. Choose from a selection of shapes (pick one that follows your natural arch) and use it to perfect your own brow.

TWEEZERS

This tool is a girl's best friend. Tweezerman or the local pharmacy will supply you – never be without it.

EYELASH CURLER

A professional make-up artist absolutely could not do without one. Even a non-make-up maven should use an eyelash curler – it adds life and body to lashes without mascara and is the one product we should never omit from our tool kit. While the heated variety work rather like an iron to keep the lashes pressed into shape for longer, standard curlers still give a perfectly satisfying result.

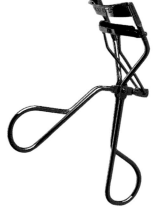

SHARP NAIL SCISSORS

These are good for trimming stray hairs, eyebrows, broken nails and many other tasks. Always keep a pair handy.

FINGERS

When applying lipsticks with your fingers, avoid the outer corners of the mouth so that you don't end up smudging the effect. Use glossy products in natural colours only in the centre of the top and bottom lips.

Cream foundation is easier to apply with your fingers than powder – just remember to blend, blend, blend, especially around the jaw line, and use less than you think you will need.

Cream blushers and eyeshadows are easier to apply with the fingertips. Keep blusher to the apples of the cheeks, and do not take eyeshadow above the crease in the eyelid.

MAKE-UP REMOVER

A good make-up remover is essential. Among the many creams, gels, mousses and wash-off cleansers on the market is a formulation for every skin type. A new addition to the range is moist wipes (ideal for travel), which will remove everything from the sheerest whisper of powder to the most stubborn patch of foundation.

WASHING YOUR BRUSHES

RUBY HAMMER, make-up artist, says: 'Always keep your brushes clean. Spray them with a liquid cleanser, or diluted shampoo, and make sure that you really wash the hairs out and rinse thoroughly. With a tissue, gently squeeze out any excess water and lay the brushes flat, with the hairy ends hanging over the edge of the table. This enables the air to circulate right through them as they dry, so they won't smell horrible when you've finished. It doesn't matter whether your brushes are sable or synthetic – I always suggest that people buy the best they can afford. Often it's best to use a mixture.'

BARE NECESSITIES

If you prefer to just brush 'n' go, your mainstay tools should be: a lip brush; a medium-sized eyeshadow brush; and a good medium-sized face brush.

SOS KIT

Elizabeth Arden's Eight Hour Cream is a wonder agent. You can use it to gloss your eyelids, heal dry patches, mend cracked lips and heels and soften cuticles. If you run out of hair gel, it can double as a styling product and, mixed with powder shadow, it makes cheek and eye products creamier and easier to apply.

OPTREX FRESH EYES IS A SISTER PRODUCT of the standard Optrex Eye Drops, just for cosmetic use. They feel refreshing, hydrating and cooling, and give your face a clearer, fresher overall look.

A MULTIPLE-PURPOSE STICK (like François Nars's Multiple). This is the staple product of modern make-up. Use on your eyes, cheeks, lips, brow bone and décolletage.

TWEEZERS – for emergency removals.

COTTON BUDS (Q-TIPS) are great for softening colour, blending and, if push comes to shove, even applying colour. A bud is also good for removing make-up, so minor mistakes do not become disasters. A much-underestimated tool.

A TRANSPARENT CONTAINER means you can stop frantically fumbling around for that missing cotton bud (Q-Tip).

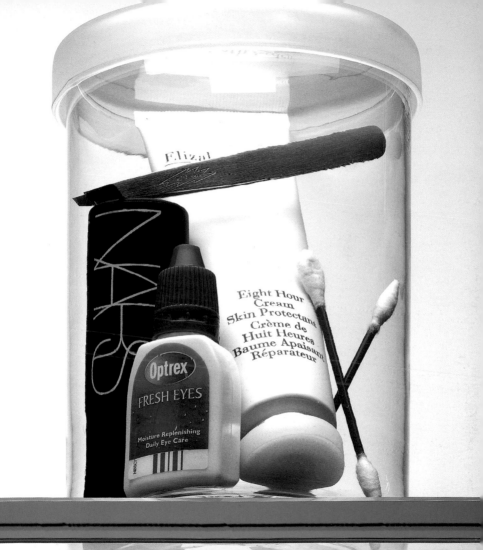

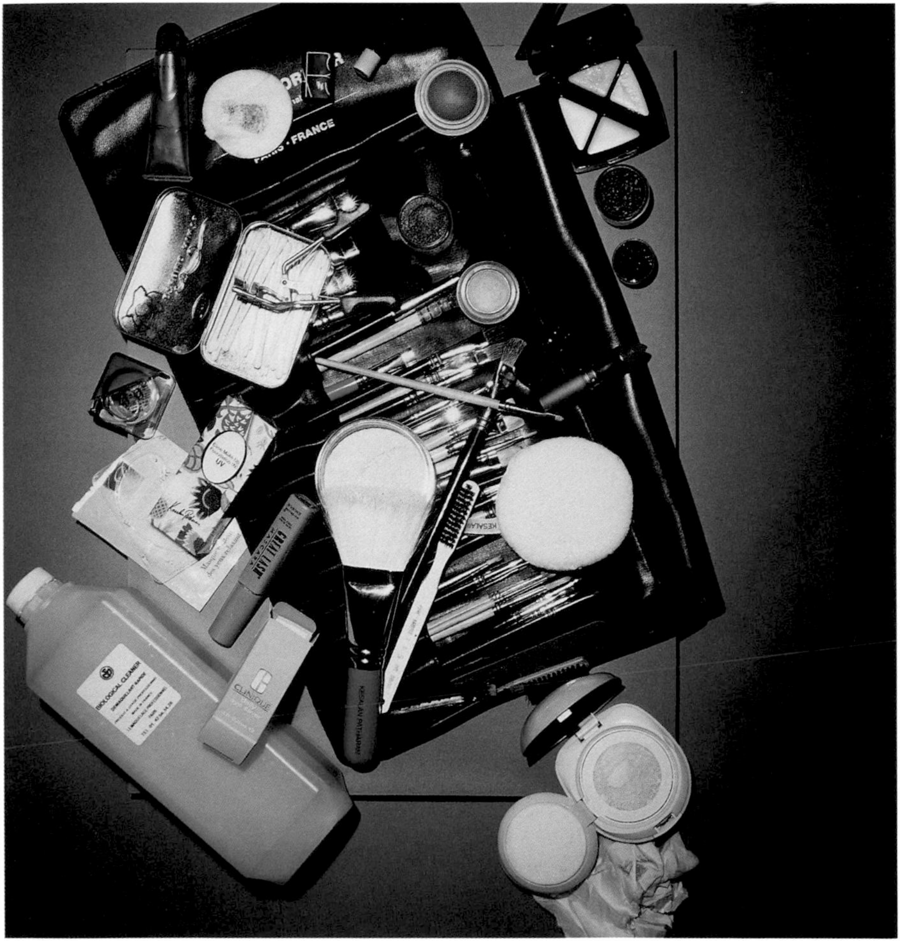
PARIS • FRANCE
UV
BIOLOGICAL CLEANER
CLINIQUE

secret weapon

(THE PROFESSIONAL MAKE-UP ARTIST)

Even if you do not possess a single make-up brush, you can still have a secret weapon in your armoury – the best and yet most often overlooked tool of all is the professional make-up artist. Not just the privilege of the model or celebrity, many make-up artists are happy to take on private work (if you are happy to pay the price, that is). And let's face it, there is something incredibly glamorous about having a professional apply your make-up – it enhances your confidence (not to mention your physical appearance) and makes an evening exciting before it even starts.

As all those who have enjoyed the professional touch will tell you, it is a revolutionary experience – the creaminess of your foundation; the smooth, unbroken texture of your perfectly blended eyelids; and the glossy pout of a mouth three times fuller than the one you grew up with are just a few of the things you can never quite achieve to a similarly high standard yourself. But as we all know, practice makes perfect, and many a canny customer has picked up tricks of the trade while having her make-up done. How to pluck your eyebrows, or disguise a blemish, and exactly where to put that blusher are all secrets to which you will become privy.

Your own technique will improve immeasurably – as long as you do not feel so relaxed that you actually fall asleep.

So how do you go about finding a make-up artist? Word of mouth is often the best route, but if this fails to deliver agencies are there to help. The next time you flick through Vogue, check the make-up artist/agency credits at the side of the page – it is quite possible that the artist whose work you like does private work. If he or she is not available, the agent will be happy to suggest an alternative.

A word of warning – professional makeovers can become addictive. At prices that will set you back a meal for two at a chichi restaurant, looking a million dollars may well end up costing it.

1 Be adventurous and prepared to change: remember that the make-up artist sees you with an objective eye and will know how to show your colouring and bone structure to their best advantage. The purple eyeshadow you feel you simply cannot live without may actually do no favours for your complexion – so prepare to be told a few home truths.

2 Never be scared to voice your pet hates – it is vital that you love the outcome, after all. Just because teenage models are parading the catwalk with 'Mazola eyelids', it doesn't necessarily mean that you want to, however 'in' the look.

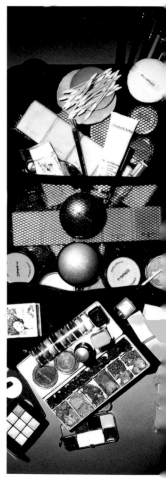

3 Maintain your confidence in your own point of view. If the acid balance in your skin always makes red lipstick turn blue, it is vital that you warn the make-up artist about this – after all, nobody knows your skin like you do.

4 Opting for a trial run is time consuming, not to mention costly, but no client worth her agency fee would contemplate embarking on a makeover without putting aside five minutes just to run through her objectives.

5 Revealing the contents of your make-up bag and the slip dress you intend to wear that night (every colour reflects light differently on to your face) are other helpful indicators of your taste and personality. You may well want to look like a Hollywood siren – but imagine your satisfaction when the siren still looks like you even after the makeover.

6 Remember that the make-up artist is so called for a reason. With years of experience on photographic shoots, he or she will understand the crucial interplay of light on the canvas of your face. Pictures give memories that last for ever, so have some taken to reap a long-term reward from your investment.

7 Invest in a proper lesson with a professional make-up artist. You will pick up tips every step of the way, ensuring the benefits won't be washed away with your make-up.

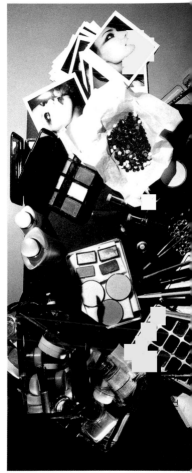

editing your make-up shelf

When did you last clean out your make-up drawer? If I am right in my guess, probably never. Scrummage right to the back, and it's more than likely you'll find a roll-on cherry lip gloss from the 1970s, a blue mascara from 1983, and a half-used bottle of Poison from whenever. While all women have an inexplicable tendency to hoard cosmetics ('I won't throw away that item just in case I need it one day'), the time has come to throw out the past and embrace the future. Remember that all good things must come to an end, and that includes your stock of old make-up.

Thanks to recent European rulings, every cosmetic item sold must now come complete with a comprehensive list of ingredients. Sell-by dates are there for a reason (even products that are crammed full of preservatives do not stay fresh for ever), and to ignore them means putting the state of your skin at risk. While out-of-date fragrance is easy to spot (the musty smell is unmistakable), other products require sharper editing. Face cream, body lotion and conditioner all thicken slowly over time, and this can easily go unnoticed.

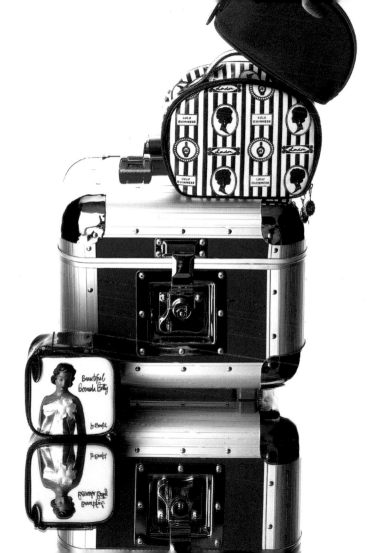

To keep your creams as fresh as your complexion, discard any jar that has been open for three months. When investing in skincare, remember that buying big can ultimately prove to be a false economy (the pot will often gone off well before you reach the bottom). Size is not everything when it comes to lotions and potions, and sharp climatic change has a detrimental effect on all cosmetic products. Cabin pressure wreaks havoc on your skin creams, so always try to decant your favourite items before you board the plane.

As any true cosmetics junkie will tell you, editing colour out of your make-up bag takes a real exercise of willpower – after all, when it comes to making faces, choice is everything. So if, like me, you find that it is impossible to pass a cosmetics counter without splashing out on 'a little something', here is one small piece of advice. Before you buy a pistachio blusher, use the tester at the counter – I find the startled expression on strangers' faces an immediate curb to my desire to spend.

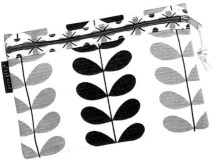

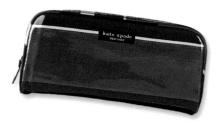
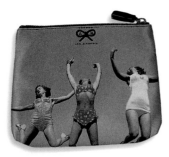

MAKE-UP TRAVEL BAGS

Given half the chance and twice the budget I would indulge in a whole luggage-line of make-up containers – not because I own an extortionate amount of products, but simply because I find the delectable array of little bags and large boxes irresistible. And with fashion infiltrating every aspect of our lifestyle, chic designer bags are here to stay. There are also a wide variety of clever make-up bags that have been especially designed to travel well. The best include:

1 Multipocketed make-up rolls on a hanger. These mean you can store every item of skincare and make-up in the same place, and just whip the roll out of your case and into your cupboard or closet as soon as you arrive at your destination.

2 Transparent make-up pouches in different sizes. Especially for the beach, they enable you to find your suncream or hair scrunchies in milliseconds and end those fruitless searches for missing items.

TIP Remember to tape down the lid of anything creamy. This will prevent messy accidents in your luggage.

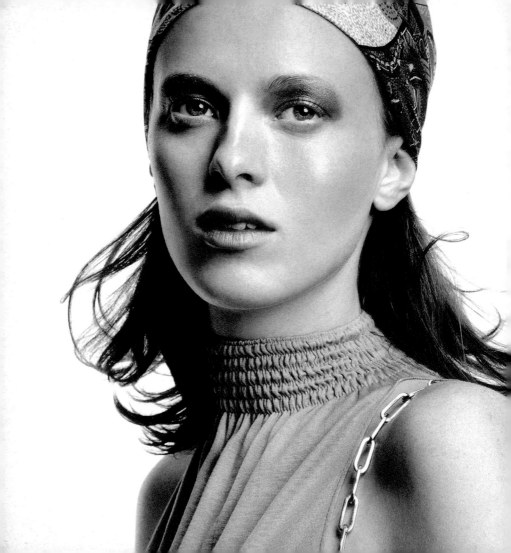

3 foundation

'Always start with a little foundation
and build it up. You can always add more.'
Ruby Hammer, make-up artist

G one are the days when a slather of uni-shade panstick saw everyone from Snow White to Pocahontas through the ABC of foundation application. Whereas once all we wanted was a way to camouflage our complexions, today's bases are cleverly concocted to enhance our natural skin tone, rather than disguise it. With the arrival of 'no make-up make-up' (and yes, every woman worth her make-up sponge has heard of it), technology has transcended anything we once thought possible – light-reflecting (rejuvenating), light-responsive (day-to-night wear) and photochromic (for when you get caught on Kodak) particles mean we can escape the ravages of time for an evening, or even for a picture. No wonder that of all the panoply of cosmetic paints and potions which entice us, foundation is the most vital to get right.

Just look upon your face as an artist's canvas – without a proper base coat, the superficial varnish will soon chip and flake. A superior foundation will make sure the top coats you apply glide on smoothly and, with a bit of luck, stay put.

More an extension of your skincare routine than a camouflage device, today's foundation comes turbo-injected with up-to-date technology. Sun protection, moisturizers, anti-ageing ingredients (such as antioxidant vitamin E), and collagen and elastin boosters (to make you look younger) are added to the colour and coverage of the modern base, combining to make a good foundation the most multipurpose product on the market. Far from impairing the skin, the modern base improves it and, most importantly, contains ingredients that allow the skin to breathe while still protecting it from environmental damage and pollution.

Years of research and development in laboratories have given us the ability to obtain a cosmetic wash-off equivalent of a new skin: these bases often contain a lower pigment concentration than a standard foundation, which allows colour to glide on without creating a solid look. And because of recent umbrella takeovers of smaller make-up houses by the skincare giants, up-to-date technology and cutting-edge ideas are more accessible.

However, the most difficult part of the foundation equation still seems to be finding exactly the right product for you. The endless choice of texture and colour is enough to confuse even the most sophisticated make-up maven, but understanding your skin type and tone is crucial to picking the right one.

Colour choice is the prime determinant as to whether you end up with a faultless complexion, or a less than convincing mask effect. The golden rule when choosing your foundation is to match it to the skin colour around your neck as exactly as possible – after all, this is the area it will need to blend into. But remember that this skin is usually fractionally darker than the skin on your face itself.

With many major houses now incorporating colours for black and Asian skins into their range, the colour choice is colossal, which means that the list of 'do nots' in foundation selection is becoming as long as the list of 'dos'.

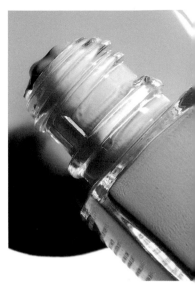

choosing a foundation

FACE FIRST

1 Never make a colour decision in artificial light. This is deceptive, and the colour can look totally different in daylight.

2 Never choose a foundation shade that is dark enough to look like a suntan.

3 Do not use a pink-based foundation to try to make yellow-toned skin look pinker, or vice versa. Instead, choose a foundation that matches your skin and let your colour cosmetics do the work afterwards.

4 Always let a colour sit on your skin for a while before you decide to purchase it. The acid balance of your skin may change the colour over time – and end up not being the right shade for your skin tone.

5 If you are not a dab hand with foundation, applying liquid coverage with a damp sponge (make sure all the excess liquid is squeezed out first) is the best way to get even coverage. Fingertip application can result in a streaky finish if you are not extra careful.

'Skin tone determines what looks best. When it comes to foundation, choose a colour that matches the skin along the jaw. That way it blends into the neck without leaving a line of demarcation. If the skin is too ruddy, use something with a yellow base to neutralize the redness. If the skin is too olive, I suggest bringing in colours like pinks or plums in the blush or lips to brighten the face. A foundation that is too pink does not look good on olive skin.'

Robin Siegel, chief make-up artist for *Friends* and celebrity make-up artist with Fred Segal Beauty, Los Angeles

6 It is important to keep the true texture of the skin, so always try to keep make-up layers to a minimum. For instance, do not use foundation around the eye area if you know that you will also be using concealer there. Apply foundation only where you genuinely need it.

FOUNDATIONS FOR ETHNIC SKINS

As a result of changing demographics and a big increase in interracial relationships, most well-known make-up brands now cater for a wide range of skin types. Where once if you had anything but the pink-toned skin of an English rose you had to seek out specialist brands to suit your colouring, today's inclusive vision of beauty means that all the major players are increasing their bases to cover an entire spectrum of skin tones – MAC and Prescriptives to name but two.

Thanks to striking and unusual models such as Devon Aoki and Alec Wek, modern make-up is rapidly embracing and revelling in our genetic differences. Old-fashioned make-up 'rules' based around our colouring, rather than on our personal preference, now seem positively archaic. With custom-blended foundation already available from higher-end product brands, it will surely not be very long before even standard bases go the couture route.

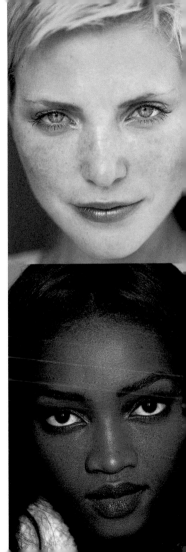

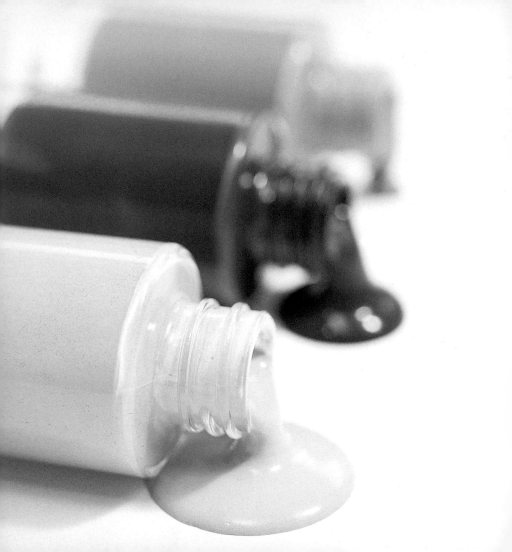

foundation textures

Consistency, as well as colour, counts, when you want to get back to bases. There is no point in creating a thick, matt mask in exactly the right beige after all. Thanks to technology, foundations now reflect light so successfully that they almost look three dimensional. This gives the modern base all the appearance of natural skin – an illusion which always escaped its predecessors. Considering we all have a unique canvas to work with, it makes sense that we have an individual make-up tailored to our personal needs. While we have a plethora of products to choose from, future foundation will certainly become bespoke, as the consumer will soon demand tailor-made texture as well as colour. However, selecting the right shade of foundation is only the beginning: transferring the product from bottle to cheek correctly is what will make or break your look. Make-up artist François Nars says: 'I meet many women who wear too much foundation. It's one of the biggest make-up problems today. There is a huge skincare movement right now, and women are taking care of their faces, so they don't need so much coverage. But as a result, some women end up not wearing anything at all, which is not good either. You have to be able to adapt to modernity and change.'

'The whole reason I wear make-up is to make my skin look smooth. For me beauty is all about a healthy, flawless complexion. I have found that foundation is the surest way to get the smooth skin I want.'

Bobbi Brown, make-up guru

SHEER FOUNDATION

A whisper of sheer foundation, dexterously applied, gives us the complexion we wish we were blessed with naturally. It usually contains silicones, which make it glide and give a soft appearance without looking oily. Used sparingly, it cannot be detected on the skin and imparts a very natural look. There are no rules about where to apply foundation – use it where you need it and blend it in carefully.

OIL-BASED FOUNDATION

This works wonders on the dry and flaky. However, a few canny tricks should be mastered to get the most from your foundation. Oil-based foundations can be slightly heavy, so add a few drops of toner to the bottle before you start – this will counteract the oil in the bottle and make your application even more sheer.

CREAM FOUNDATION

This looks lovely on more mature skins as it is smooth, milky, and kind on surface lines and wrinkles. It gives a natural-looking finish while still providing that confidence-boosting coverage.

MATT FOUNDATION

Matt foundation always needs to be applied very quickly and blended thoroughly as it does not contain any oil, so dries out the moment it touches the skin. It is great for Mediterranean skin types with oily T-zones, as it stays shine-free for longer than other foundations. But to avoid an unnaturally heavy finish it should always be applied with a very light hand to a complexion that has already been correctly moisturized.

LIGHT-REFLECTING FOUNDATION

This contains specially-shaped particles that reflect light off the skin to give it a youthful appearance. It is appropriate for young girls who want to obtain a 'dewy' complexion and for older women wishing to draw attention away from lines and wrinkles.

LIGHT-RESPONSIVE FOUNDATION

Revolutions in modern technology have delivered this foundation which contains pigments that are light sensitive, meaning they respond differently to natural and electric light, and change to maintain a 'true' colour in either.

COMPACT FOUNDATION

Powder and foundation in one, this is very easy to apply with a sponge and is the 'one-stop shopping' of foundation. Applied with a light hand, compact foundation can appear very natural; heavy-handed application, though, leads to a mask-like finish.

HIGHLIGHTING STICK

Not foundation as such, but these sticks, which are superb for highlighting the face or body, add a sexy glow to selected areas and can be used either alone or in conjunction with other foundation products. François Nars makes fabulous multipurpose versions.

TINTED MOISTURIZER

Fantastic for enhancing a suntan or for regular use by those blessed with flawless skin, tinted moisturizer gives minimal

PRIMERS

Magic base coat or wily marketing ploy? While anyone with as much sense as money might be loathe to pay for a truly invisible product, those with uneven complexions will find them worth a try. While primers do not actually improve skin in the long term, they enhance its appearance by tightening pores and boosting elasticity for an evening. The way they work is two-fold: firstly, they stop the skin from 'drinking' your foundation (goodbye end-of-evening patchy look) and, secondly, they stop foundation absorbing too much sebum. In short, they create a velvety surface for your base to glide on, giving a natural glow. Unlike moisturizer under foundation, a primer stays put.

Chantecaille's Real Skin provides the most natural looking coverage. Colour is suspended in a gel so it glides on easily as well as giving a brighter, sparkling complexion. Future Skin – the alternative to Real Skin for those with greasier complexions – is an even lighter formulation that is oil-free. Estée Lauder's Spotlight boasts revolutionary optical technology called 'specular reflection'. As the foundation contains many layered particles, hundreds of reflections occur simultaneously and prevent the eye from focusing on any one layer. This creates a sense of depth and a youthful glow. Estée Lauder's light-responsive make-up, Revelation, was not only light diffusing (that is, it reflected light to divert attention from lines and wrinkles) but light responsive, too. Because of the photochromic pigment it contained, the foundation changed colour in different lights, meaning that it looked just as natural in broad daylight as it did in a candle-lit evening glow.

coverage and adds a smidgen of colour to your complexion. Be sure to blend in well to avoid a patchy finish.

GEL FOUNDATION

In one of the newest additions to the foundation family, colour pigments are suspended in a gel-like formulation that glides on easily, absorbs well, and leaves you with sheer, natural-looking coverage. Try those by François Nars and Chantecaille.

PEARLIZED UNDERCOAT

This can be used on its own for a wet-look finish or as a highlighter. Worn under foundation, it adds a subtle shimmer to your complexion. Lancôme's Maquisuperbe is my favourite.

MAKE-UP ARTISTS' TOP TIPS FOR APPLYING FOUNDATION PERFECTLY

'Don't let yourself in for a nasty surprise. Always check your make-up in more than one mirror, and in more than one light, before you go out. Make sure that your neck and bosom do not stand out in stark contrast to your face.'
MAGGIE HUNT

'What you have to remember when you're covering such a huge area of your face is that it's not a flat surface. It has nooks and crannies, blood vessels and contours – you need to pick tools which can deal with all these areas.'
RUBY HAMMER

'I prefer a non-oily foundation, even on dry skin, because you can always moisturize first. Foundation applied lightly can even out any skin tone and hide blotchiness. It shouldn't feel like a mask. If it does, you are wearing too much.'
KEVYN AUCOIN

'Older women often think that their foundation has changed because it doesn't suit them any more. What they don't realize is that often it is their complexion that has changed, for example become paler, as they have aged. It is important not to get stuck in a foundation rut.'
STEPHEN GLASS

'Forget sponges. I always prefer to apply make-up with my fingers; it helps you reach places that sponges never can, and avoids streaking.'
MARY GREENWELL

'I always like to put make-up on in natural daylight. This way you won't get any nasty surprises.'
BOBBI BROWN

skin perfectors

To the non-professional eye, these pastel-coloured skin products can seem somewhat scary. However, they work wonders to disguise uneven pigment, or to calm down the appearance of high coloration. Use them sparingly underneath your foundation, and you will be amazed at the results. My personal favourite is Lancôme's Palette Pro, which contains concealers to cover every predicament, and comes packaged in an easy-to-use compact.

GREEN counteracts redness. Use on blotchy patches and also to disguise broken veins.

YELLOW can seem a godsend after a late night because it has an 'anti-fatigue' action that counteracts dark circles under the eyes.

LILAC gives a welcome lift to sallow skin and helps to eradicate a dull complexion.

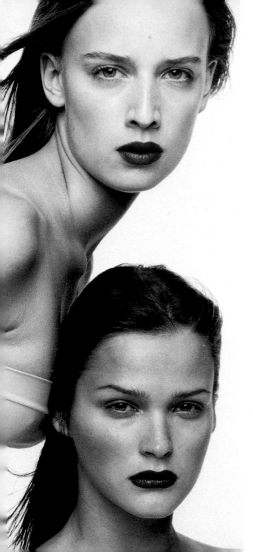

BARBARA DALY'S FOUNDATION TIPS

1 The best way to choose your perfect colour is to blend a small amount of foundation along your jaw line – the right colour will 'disappear' into your skin.

2 Even if your skin is good enough not to need foundation, you may still benefit from a little, just to even out any discoloration on specific areas such as around the nose or chin.

3 Remember that it is always best to start with a little foundation and build up coverage slowly, rather than put on too much and have to remove it.

4 If your skin changes shade throughout the year (that is, it looks paler in winter than it does in summer) and you fall between colours, buy two shades of liquid foundation and mix a little together on the back of your hand before applying it to the face.

application

Getting your base absolutely right is essential to the success of your overall look, so mastering the art of application is (almost) everything here. Resist the temptation to be overzealous in the foundation department, as fashion's movement towards a far more natural look (not to mention the technology that renders new foundations as convincing as your own bare skin) means less is always more. Make-up artist Dick Page explains: 'You should always use a very light hand when applying foundation. Remember to pay particular attention to your skin tone, and only use product where you actually need to apply it. Always work in natural daylight, and remember that when it comes to buying foundations, opting for a cheap and cheerful product is often a false economy. You will get more for your money if you stick to a top-end product from, say, Lancôme or Lauder. Tinted moisturizer is underrated, but great if you've got an even skin tone.'

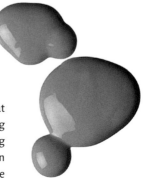

It is not just what you use, but the way that you use it that counts. For those who prefer to use their fingertips, avoiding the temptation to slap on foundation as if it were shaving foam is key. To make sure you do not end up looking like an extra from *Cabaret*, mix a little foundation with your favourite moisturizer before you apply it, which will help thin it out a little and aid a smooth application. Use your fingers to get into all the bony areas (around your nose, under your chin), and never forget to blend, particularly around the jaw line. Foundation sponges are great, as they absorb the base, making it almost impossible to apply too much. Stick to synthetic sponges (my favourites are by MAC, Shu Uemura and Ruby & Millie), as these absorb the product more evenly and lead to an ultimately smoother finish. Make sure your sponges are slightly damp (not wet, as this will make the foundation streaky) before you start. While there is no need to apply foundation everywhere (today's bases should be indistinguishable from areas of natural skin), it is true that it does help other make-up products glide on more easily. One area I always prime with base is my eyelids (nothing supplies a smoother base for non-chip, non-flake eyeshadow), while just a dab of base over the lips lets you create a cleaner lip line and makes sure your lipstick does not leave the party before you do.

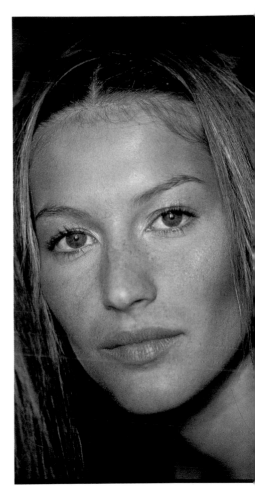

concealer

'A good concealer is the secret of the universe,' according to make-up guru Bobbi Brown, and it is easy to see why. Just the right colour, in just the right texture, and you would need a magnifying glass to prove that Mother Nature did not bless you with a perfect canvas. Just the wrong shade, in just the wrong texture, and you will draw attention to those blemishes you sought to disguise. With a multitude of products available in every tone and texture (tubes of cream, liquids with sponge-tip applicators, simple sticks and harder 'cake' compacts), there is something for everyone – the trick is knowing how to use the right product in the right place.

When it comes to covering spots and blemishes, use a hard concealer to make sure your camouflage stays put. 'Always apply it with a fine-tipped brush,' says make-up doyenne Maggie Hunt, 'and place it exactly on top of the blemish, not on the surrounding skin.' If there is not a concealer to match your foundation, opt for one a shade lighter. A concealer that is even one shade too dark will serve only to highlight an imminent eruption.

The under-eye bags that follow late nights and excessive drinking are virtually impossible to conceal (although cold tea bags have been found to work wonders in reducing puffiness), but there are a few tricks that will help disguise them. Using a creamy, liquid concealer (this blends most successfully into delicate under-eye skin), pat tiny dots around the orbital bone. Using your fingertips, gently blend the concealer in until it disappears. Products with light-reflecting particles, such as Yves Saint Laurent's miracle-working Touche Éclat, knock years off by radically diminishing shadows in seconds. Used as a highlighter on the brow bone, or down the creases that run from the sides of your nose to your lips, it will brighten your complexion and magically rejuvenate your appearance.

The golden rule of concealer, remember, is never to sabotage the desired effect by using the wrong product in the wrong location – you would not treat a headache with a cough lozenge, would you? Hard concealers used around crow's-feet will crumble and look unsightly, while a product that is too soft will slip off a blemish and end up on your collar. For me, the confidence boost created by the right camouflage is priceless.

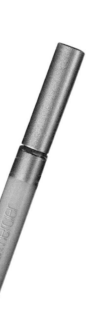

powder

Once almost a dirty word among make-up mavens, powder has come back with a vengeance. However, today's take on powder has little or nothing to do with the talcum-powder dusting of yesterday. Less is certainly more when it comes to both the colour (as translucent as possible) and the texture (as sheer as possible) of the modern product. Whether it is loose or pressed, powder works as an invisible fixer that helps colour cosmetics brush on easily and smoothly over foundation without blotching or creasing. Dusted loosely under the eyes before eye make-up is applied, powder acts as a magnet for any falling shadow and can be swept away with a soft brush without leaving your face streaked with colour.

With powder, the means is just as important as the end. Using the right tool for application will make a surprising difference to the quality of the finish. The more soft and voluminous the brush and the more natural the fibre, the better. Satisfyingly chunky to hold, a powder brush by Shu Uemura will set you back the price of an expensive meal, but console yourself by thinking how much prettier you will look as a result the next time you go out.

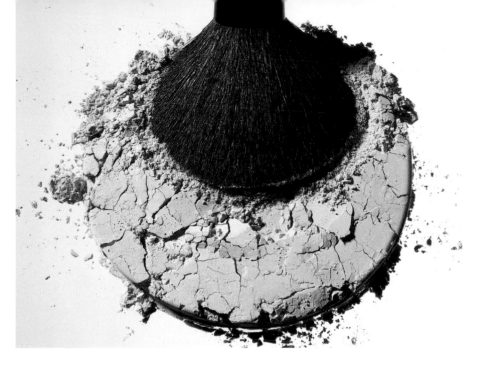

For achieving the desired barely-there effect, application is key. After dipping your brush into the magic dust, gently blow any excess powder off the bristles. If your technique is restrained, a little powder placed under your eyes, down the bridge of your nose and onto the tip of your chin is a wonderful form of highlighting. Best of all, most men still associate foundation with a pre-historic panstick look, so if you apply your base flawlessly and finish with a whisper of sheer powder, he will never know you are wearing any.

bases

HOLIDAY BASE

A sun-kissed complexion sends confidence soaring sky-high, but getting your make-up right as well maximizes your holiday appeal.

1 In hot weather, your skin looks and behaves differently, and tends to sweat more. As a result, less is definitely more in the make-up equation.

2 As your skin tans, you need more colour but less coverage from your base. A tinted moisturizer is brilliant for enhancing a natural suntan. 'A good way to test a tinted moisturizer is down the centre panel of your nose,' says Millie of Ruby & Millie. 'This way you will see if it is going to settle well around the pores.'

3 Always use a product with a sunscreen, both at home and on holiday, as damage from UVA rays accounts for the majority of visible premature skin ageing.

4 The sun tends to dry up blemishes and even out a patchy complexion, so apply coverage only where you really need it.

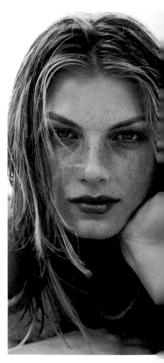

5 Never travel without a good concealer. Even if your honeyed skin looks fabulous, everyone will benefit from a little camouflage, lightly applied in just the right places. A dual concealer (such as those by Laura Mercier and Ruby & Millie) allows you to blend two shades as your suntan deepens, so you can mix exactly the colour you need.

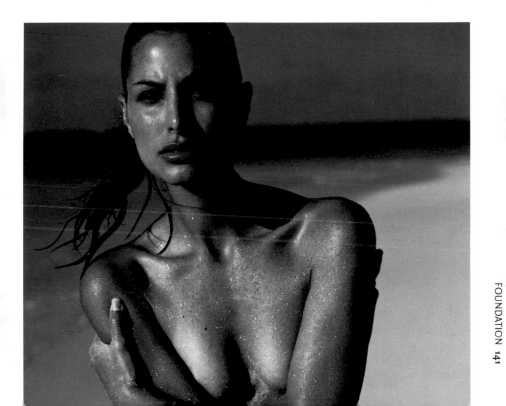

EVERYDAY BASE

Avoid the base mistake – do not just slap on the same old product in the same old places day after day. Take a moment to look at yourself when you wake up in the morning. Our lifestyle plays a major role in the way that our skin behaves and, as our epidermis is a living organism, it changes with the weather, levels of pollution and our fluctuating hormone cycles. Pay close attention to your skin's needs, and apply only what you need where you need it.

1 Before you even consider applying foundation, make sure you are using the right skincare so that you start off with as clear a complexion as possible.

2 Then assess the condition of your skin. Premenstrually, for example, it may appear spottier,and require special care.

3 Even if your skin looks wonderful, it is possible to enhance its flawless look further by using concealer a couple of shades lighter than the skin underneath your eyes (to disguise any dark circles) and dabbing some at the sides of your nose (to counteract redness).

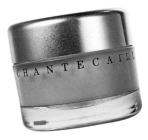

4 A mere whisper of powder is a superb alternative to a base for those fortunate enough to be blessed with an even skin tone. Translucent powder creates an imperceptible veil that not only 'finishes off' your face, but also acts as a delicate mop to soak up any excess sebum.

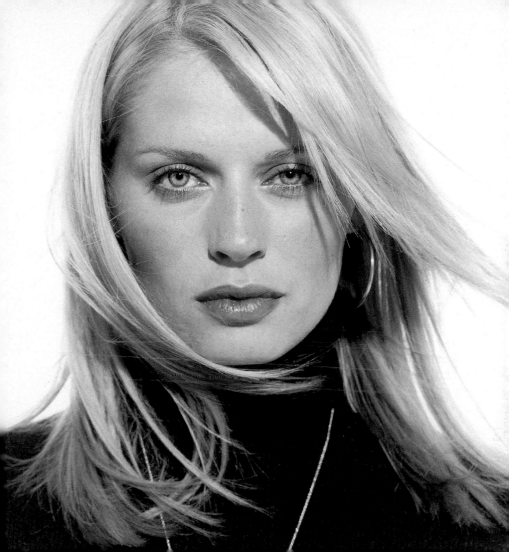

5 Avoid heavy-duty liquid foundations for use during the day. Instead, a compact foundation, used lightly, offers enough coverage for most people and looks natural when not overapplied. It also fits conveniently into your handbag. Stick to oil-free products for daytime use even if you have dry skin (you can always compensate with a rich moisturizer), as these tend to stay put for longer periods and thus serve you better throughout the day.

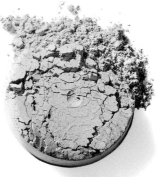

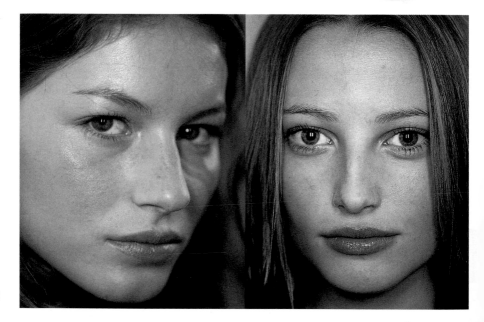

EVENING BASE

Looking your best is always important, but it is never more so than when you anticipate a great night out. Although the softer light of evening is kinder to our complexions, most of us spend more time worrying about our 'social' face than our work one. To make sure you always make an entrance wherever you go, here are a few helpful hints:

1 Use a fluid foundation at night. The softer electric lighting means you can get away with heavier coverage than during the day, but don't go overboard.

2 For the evening, use a powder blush. Cream blushers create an extremely natural effect that looks fine in daylight, but they can fade away to nothing when combined with a fluid foundation.

3 Remember that highlighters are excellent for enhancing your features at night – darker shades will make chosen areas of the face recede, while lighter colours will push them forwards. Used carefully, they can redefine your jaw line, reduce the appearance of your nose, enlarge your eyes and really make them stand out, and even create a generous cleavage. The darker the shade of powder you use, the deeper the contour will look. One tip is that, if you use a shader, you must always balance it with a highlighter somewhere else. Always select a reasonably stiff, angled brush to shade and highlight.

4 If you cannot master the art of shading and highlighting (don't give up too soon, as practice really does make perfect), changing the shape of your eyebrows will have a dramatic effect on the appearance of your face. Lengthening them with an eye pencil, for example, will immediately make your jaw look narrower. Remember to apply foundation all the way down the sides of your face, as this will help to keep your new eyebrows in place.

5 At night, always, always apply foundation to your eyelids. It is the best way to hold your eye make-up in place.

6 Just as with your eyes, applying foundation to your lips will increase the quality and lifespan of your lipstick.

DEWY BASE

The world of fashion has catapulted the 'dewy' complexion to the forefront of our consciousness. However, achieving a moist, appealing complexion, as opposed to one that looks as though you have just given yourself a facial with olive oil, takes practice and just the right products. Make-up guru Ruby Hammer, of Ruby & Millie, has made up hundreds of celebrity faces. She lets us in on how to achieve the perfect dewy look:

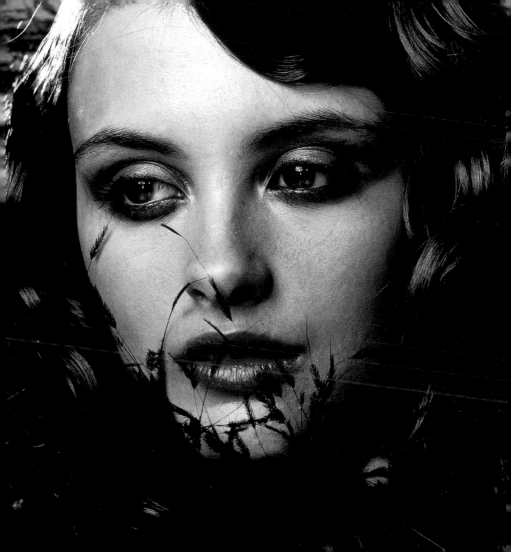

RUBY HAMMER'S TIPS
FOR A DEWY COMPLEXION

1 Look for a base with a low powder concentration (both Shu Uemura and Givenchy make good ones).

2 Remember that the water content of a dewy foundation may evaporate and leave an oily residue on your skin, so apply it at the last minute, and do not expect it to last for hours.

3 Bear in mind that, while a 'dewy' foundation reflects light and thus lends the skin a youthful glow, it is a double-edged sword, as it has a habit of sliding. This can leave more mature skins looking either too naked or somewhat greasy.

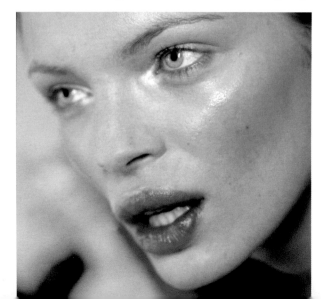

OPEN PORES

Visible pores are the bane of the olive-skinned. Usually scattered across the nose and cheeks, they can make the sufferer feel as though she has open craters on her face. Products that are too creamy accentuate the problem and can lead to spots (the open pores absorb them), but products that are too dry do not sit comfortably on the skin. Although it is difficult to eradicate open pores entirely, there are ways to minimize them for an evening out:

1 Invest in a primer. This will tighten the pores before you apply your foundation.

2 Steam your face regularly to remove blackheads and blockages, then pat it with a cool towel to shrink the pores once they are cleansed. Never use either boiling or freezing water, as you will risk developing broken capillaries.

3 Before an evening out, apply a toner. The astringent quality of the product will superficially tighten pores, although you should avoid toning regularly as it dries out the skin.

4 Use pore-cleansing strips across the nose. These water-activated adhesive strips draw dirt up to the surface of the skin and remove it as you peel them off. Resist the temptation to use them more than a couple of times a week.

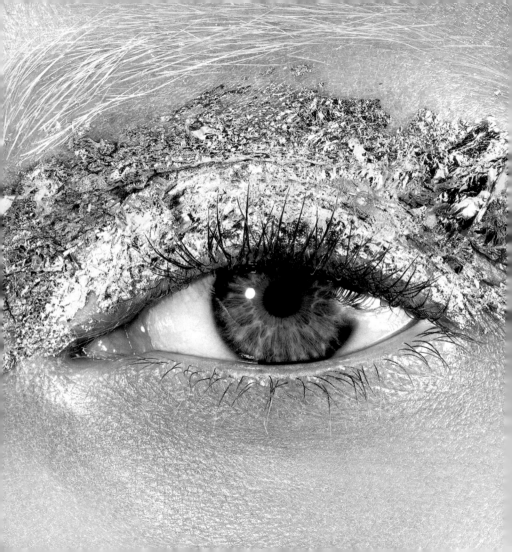

4

eyes

'The eyes have no real limitations. Each shape you create, whether with shadows, pencils or liner, can take you into completely different realms.'
Kevyn Aucoin, make-up artist

S top hiding behind those Prada shades and accept that your eyes always give away your age. No matter how hard we work at keeping other areas of our body looking young, telltale 'laughter lines' will insist on fanning out visibly at the corners of our eyes. And it does not stop there. The onset of crow's-feet means we are only the twinkling of an eye away from a pair of crepey eyelids (the sort that not even one of Stila's glossiest shadows will stick to), making it even harder to wear make-up, just when we need it most.

But before you take the drastic action of giving up laughing altogether, think about how hard the eye area actually works. Considering that eye muscles move on average an astounding 100,000 times a day, it is not altogether surprising that the eye area is particularly prone to premature ageing. Add to this the fact that the skin around the eye is only 0.5 mm (1/32 in) thick and roughly half the density of the skin on the rest of your face, and you will swiftly realize that maintaining a pair of youthful-looking peepers is going to require a substantial outlay, both in time and money.

Of course, not everybody over the age of 29 walks around with under-eye bags larger than a Fendi tote. Among the array of anti-ageing products which saturate the market are some highly effective lotions and potions that protect the eye area from dehydration, UV rays and atmospheric damage, as well as smoothing out the appearance of surface lines and wrinkles.

'If you wake up with puffy eyes, chances are the moisturizer you used the night before is too rich or you applied too much. A trick for covering dark circles is to use a concealer with a warm peach tone to neutralize the bluish tone of the dark circle.'
Robin Siegel, chief make-up artist for *Friends* and celebrity make-up artist with Fred Segal Beauty, Los Angeles

Available in different forms (creams, gels, capsules, mousses and masks) and for every age group and skin type, today's eye products are more effective than ever before. Modern thinking embraces an alliance of both hi-tech and natural ingredients in eye care, enabling the forces of science and nature to combine in the battle against premature ageing.

DID YOU KNOW?

1 That your skin gets warmer while you sleep, allowing it to absorb active ingredients more easily. That is why intensive eye treatments are best used at night.

2 That the majority of blepharoplasty or 'eye job' operations are sought by women who have spent years overapplying gel to the eye area. Unable to break down, it sits as unsightly deposits under the eye, resulting in bags that can be removed only by a plastic surgeon.

3 That using eye creams with natural ingredients is not always the gentlest way to treat the delicate skin surrounding your peepers. If you have sensitive skin, you may be allergic to live plant extracts and should opt instead for hypoallergenic products, which probably contain more chemical ingredients, but will ultimately be better for your skin type.

HORSETAIL EXTRACT to improve microcirculation and elasticity.

ROSEWATER AND CORNFLOWER to soothe and smooth.

VITAMIN B to help moisturize. (Vitamin B is now used routinely by many of the major beauty houses.)

CAMOMILE AND MALLOW to cool. (Aromatherapy company Elemis makes a marvellously refreshing eye gel – use it sparingly.)

BAGGY EYES

Eyelids with more puff than pastry are a common indication of fluid retention, which occurs when liquid waste accumulates in the delicate under-eye tissue. This is caused by the slowing down of lymph circulation, particularly overnight when the eyelids are not moving to promote drainage. Poor circulation, hormone cycles and oily skincare products all exacerbate the problem, and the only way to improve puffy eyes in the long term is to cut down on your intake of salt, caffeine and alcohol (especially red wine), and stick to a diet that is rich in fresh fruit and vegetables; drinking eight glasses of water a day also helps.

If you do not fancy changing your diet or lifestyle, there are products available that act as a poultice by drawing out excess fluid to help reduce the prominence of under-eye bags (Clarins and Estée Lauder both make effective ones). These work in much the same way as traditional remedies such as cold tea bags or cucumber slices. Tapping lightly under the eye area with an index finger for a couple of minutes also produces visible results.

DARK CIRCLES

The bluish, shadowy under-eye circles that so many of us suffer from occur when the circulation in this area slows down. As a consequence, blood pigments stagnate and are particularly visible through the fine, under-eye skin. Partly hereditary, under-eye circles can also be caused by lack of sleep and overexposure to the sun. Eye creams that contain ingredients to fight harmful free radicals and to break up the accumulation of blood cells can slightly reduce the 'blue-ringed' look if they are used regularly over a period of time.

Sadly, there is no miracle cure for under-eye circles. That said, one of the best ways to minimize the appearance of dark shadows is to pat a good liquid concealer, about two shades lighter than your foundation, around the sockets. Blend it in well, using light, feathery movements with your fingertips. Do not apply foundation in addition to concealer below the eyes, as the layering of products in this area will end up looking very unnatural.

DON'T BE BLINDED BY SCIENCE

Technological discoveries include:

OXYGEN DELIVERY SYSTEMS – the talk of LA. They infuse the fragile skin surrounding the eye area with pure oxygen molecules to breathe life back into tired eyes. (Try Lancaster's Oxygen Supply.)

ANTIOXIDANT VITAMINS A, C AND E, which will protect skin from toxin damage and keep the eye area looking young. (Skincare company Osmotics makes Anti-wrinkle Vitamin C patches, which, worn around the eye area while you sleep, use vitamin C to counter free-radical damage and collagen breakdown in the skin.)

PHYSICAL AND CHEMICAL SUNSCREENS that protect the eye area from the UV damage that leads to premature skin ageing.

COLLAGEN FIBRES, to boost the skin's elasticity.

THE MORNING AFTER

How many times have you rolled out of bed, feeling a little the worse for wear, only to be greeted by a red-eyed monster staring back at you from the mirror? Here are a few ways to look like an angel even when you have behaved like a little devil:

1 After a night of excess, sleep with an extra pillow – this prevents eye fluids from accumulating in the sockets and reduces bags.

2 Splash your face with cool water. This will immediately boost the circulation, and brighten up a slack, greyish complexion.

3 Moisturize well, especially under the eyes, where the fine skin will be dehydrated. Avoid products with known irritants such as alpha-hydroxy acids or retinoids, and rich creams that can swamp delicate under-eye skin and result in small white cysts.

4 Use some glycerine drops, which act like false tears to wash the eyes and help soothe them.

TIPS FOR TIRED EYES

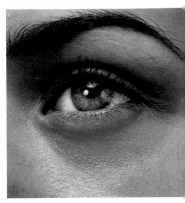

1 Steal a tip from the supermodels and use brightening eye drops to banish the red-veined look instantly. Only do this in an emergency, as these drops work by constricting the capillaries in the eye, which may come back redder with overuse.

2 If you do not have a jar of the latest wonder product to hand, slices of raw potato will reduce puffiness.

3 Crush some ice, wrap it in a handkerchief and lie with it under your eyes for as long as you can bear. This will diminish bags by constricting the blood vessels under the eyes.

4 Catch up on some sleep. This is the best way to achieve naturally bright eyes.

5 If all else fails, pretend you work in fashion or film, and wear your sunglasses inside.

WONDER PRODUCT

Yves Saint Laurent's Touche Éclat will knock years off you in milliseconds. Packaged in a 'felt-tip' applicator for easy use, this under-eye concealer contains light-reflecting particles that work as if by magic to detract attention from lines and wrinkles. There is simply nothing else like it.

CAUGHT WITH NO EYE MAKE-UP?

1 Vaseline is a miracle product. Smear it across your eyelids by itself, or mix it with powder blush to create eye shadow.

2 Bend your eyelashes back with your finger from the root, and keep them there for a few moments as the next best thing to eyelash curlers.

3 Improvize. Lipstick will double up as eyeshadow and a natural lip liner as an eyeliner.

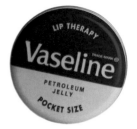

THE FRESH-EYED APPROACH

1 Make sure that you always read by a proper light, and wear glasses if you need them. This will prevent you from squinting, causing premature wrinkles to appear around the corners of your eyes.

2 Use a good eye make-up remover to take your make-up off every night. Use a gentle sweeping motion from the outside in, as this will stop you pulling the skin and stretching it.

3 Stop smoking – in tests conducted on identical twins at St Thomas's Hospital, London, those who smoked had skin that had thinned (and therefore visibly aged) by up to 40 per cent more than their non-smoking twin.

4 Use hypoallergenic eye make-up if you have sensitive skin.

eyebrows

Change your eyebrows, and you totally redefine your personality. Perhaps, above all other features, the way we shape our brows (or not) speaks volumes about the way we see ourselves and the way that others see us. Just think about it – the 'take me or leave me' attitude expressed by the babe who chooses to leave the fluff between her brows, the 'high maintenance' appearance of the girl whose brows are always perfectly arched, and the 'sex kitten' smouldering of the bleached-out bombshell express a love or hate relationship with the tweezers. Our eyebrows are the closest we get to a facial signature – just try picturing Brooke Shields or Elizabeth Taylor without their trademark pairs. While fashions for thicker or thinner brows change frequently, those who were born with a strong pair should wear them with pride, or at least think twice before plucking them into obscurity. Many a 1960s siren now regrets the pencil-thin remnants of an arc left after years of demolishing a once defined curve.

For those not blessed with naturally shaped brows, both permanent and less drastic forms of cosmetic enhancement abound. For anyone with supreme certainty about the shape and colour she requires, tattooing is a marvellous

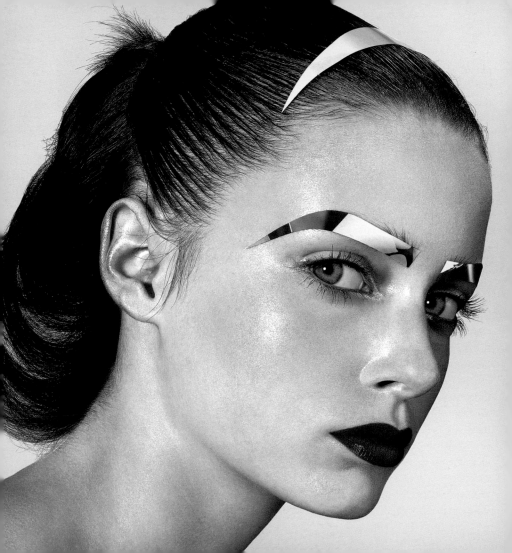

no-maintenance option. Once the inked-in brows are in place, you can forget about them for weeks – and taking the eyebrow plunge means that swimming will no longer threaten to wash two 'rainbows' down your cheek.

While bleaching or dyeing the brows to match your hair colour is vital to pulling off a natural-looking hairstyle, eyebrow pencils are another, more convenient and easy to apply method of altering your natural shade. One top tip from make-up artist Maggie Hunt is always to keep the eyebrow pencil one shade lighter than your hair colour for a convincing result.

For those who are too chicken to pluck, 'stringing' or 'threading' is a fast and relatively pain-free method of removing eyebrow hairs. Originating in Asia as a cheaper, less messy alternative to waxing, this treatment is now widely available at major beauty salons and some beauty counters in department stores. It involves a skilled therapist tweaking out hairs in a perfect curve using nothing but a piece of high-tension string.

Electrolysis is the permanent way to shapely brows, for once you have completed a course the hairs will never grow back. Costly and sometimes painful, electrolysis will save you unsightly regrowth, but limits your options should you change your mind.

Traditionalists will never be parted from their tweezers. While make-up artists, models and celebrities all swear by the Tweezerman brand, tweezer preference boils down to personal choice. As a general rule, the slanted-end type are better for gripping obstinate hairs, but, for the dextrous plucker, a pointed pair will do just fine. If you do prefer to pluck, there are a few handy hints to maximize your natural curves – only ever remove hairs from underneath the brow (spiky regrowth around the forehead looks unsightly) and avoid leaving a thick wedge of hair on the inner edges of your brows (the 'tadpole' look makes the eyes appear close set and always draws attention to your nose). (See pages 163–4 for more ways to achieve perfect brows.)

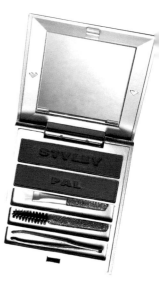

HOW TO BE HIGHBROW

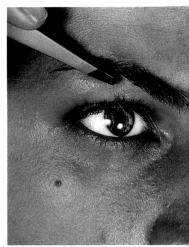

1 Eyebrows are possibly the most defining feature of the face, so tread carefully if you intend to alter them. Remember that even if you do not want to change the natural shape of your eyebrows, brushing them upwards, or flattening them with hair gel or transparent mascara will give your overall look a little extra polish, and separate the women from the girls.

2 When tweezing, always cleanse the area to be worked on with a cotton bud (Q-Tip) that has been soaked in toner first.

3 Start at the side of the brow nearest your nose and work outwards, removing a continuous line of hairs at a time. Avoid a 'tadpole' shape, which will make eyes appear close set.

4 Remember that the more you pluck away from beneath your brows, the greater the space you create for applying eye make-up.

5 Your eye shape will naturally determine what shape eyebrow suits your face best, and whether you should go really thin, or retain a slightly fuller feel.

6 Before you pluck out any stray hairs, draw your new brow shape in with white eyeliner first, to make sure you are happy with the overall outline.

7 Never pluck above your eyebrows. Instead, any unwanted growth above your perfect curve should be bleached into insignificance with some very carefully applied facial hair lightener.

8 Top make-up artist Kevyn Aucoin suggests bleaching your eyebrows up to two shades lighter than your hair colour for the most attractive and flattering finish.

9 When filling in patchy sections with an eyebrow pencil, use broken movements to keep the effect looking natural. Stick to an eyebrow pencil about one shade lighter than your brows or the new additions will always be very obvious.

10 If you want made-up brows to last a whole day, make-up artist Vincent Longo suggests 'using pencil first, and then applying matching powder shadow on top'.

11 Unfortunately, the hair regrowth that inevitably follows plucking is very noticeable on anyone whose hair colour is any shade other than flaxen (and who probably will not need to pluck in any case). Electrolysis can be painful, but because it is a permanent form of hair removal you avoid the unsightly stubble stage, and the chore of plucking from then on.

TRANSFORM YOUR EYEBROWS

Kevyn Aucoin, make-up artist, has
some advice for when you want to
change your eyebrow shape for the
evening, but without plucking:

1 Cover your natural brow with sealing wax.

2 'Paint' over the waxed brow with a fixer
   and let it dry.

3 Cover the sealed brow with foundation.

4 Lightly dust with translucent powder.

5 Draw on your new brow shape with an
   eyebrow pencil.

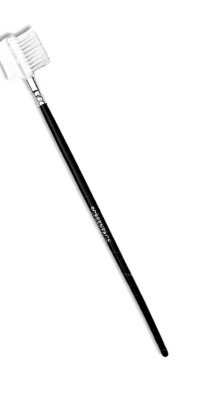

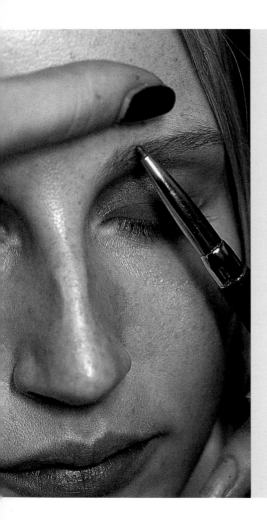

RUBY HAMMER, co-founder of Ruby & Millie Cosmetics, is an expert at achieving perfect brows and turning bushbabies into super babes.

1 Find the highest part of your eyebrow. This is where it should arch. From this point on, it should gradually slope downwards.

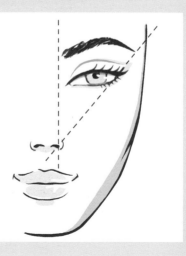

Ruby Hammer's brow-shaping tips

2 Hold a pencil flat along the side of your nose. This is where your eyebrow should start. Then move it to the outer corner of your eye – this is where it should end.

3 Do not overpluck. Just a few hairs plucked from under your brow can dramatically change your look. If you are having your brows tweezed professionally, ask if you can remain standing – you look different lying down.

4 Always pluck hairs one line at a time from underneath the brow, then stand back and glance at your overall look before plucking another line.

5 Use colour to fill in gaps and create uniformity and texture. Don't be heavy handed when you apply it.

6 When you dye your hair, remember to match your eyebrows to your new colour. Nothing looks worse than a blonde bombshell with dark eyebrows.

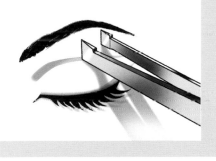

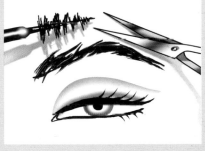

eyelashes

Even the most resolute make-up minimalist wants a great set of eyelashes. Framed by some well-groomed fringing, your eyes look sultry and seductive – without them you risk looking like an albino rabbit. While tinting and perming are good wash-proof ways to attain a perfect pair of flutterers, for those who are happy to settle for what nature gave them, mascara, eyelash curlers, and even nylon falsies and some rubber gum are enough to create luxuriant lashes.

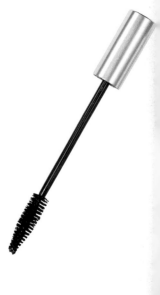

One of the most important yet most neglected tools of the trade is the eyelash curler. No professional make-up artist or model would be caught without theirs, yet most of us shy away from this medieval-looking instrument of torture. Used carefully it is harmless enough, but always go gently near the eyelid, as clamping down hard on your sensitive skin can prove somewhat painful. As any make-up maven will tell you, once you have mastered the art of squeezing gently along the length of your lashes, you will never go anywhere without a perfectly groomed set of lashes again. Keep the pressure the same along the whole length of your lashes, or, rather than a gentle curve, you could end up with a right angle.

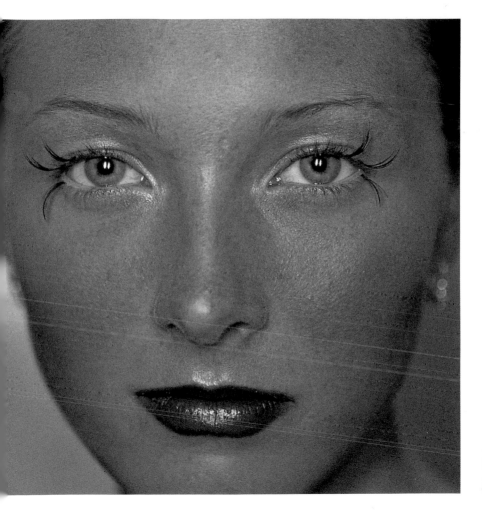

Of course, there are products to suit every whim and need, and thanks to technological advancement, you can call upon lengthening, thickening, transparent, darkening, colouring, conditioning and waterproof mascaras from every brand name under the sun. When applying mascara, there are a few key hints which, properly mastered, will ensure optimum results. Above all, never apply it directly to the roots: always sweep upwards in a gentle curve and comb between the lashes before applying a second coat if you do not want to resemble Spider-Man.

FALSE LASHES

A set of falsies can enhance any girl's natural curves – especially in the eyelash department. Now that false lashes are no longer only available in a totally solid rainbow-shaped curve, those in the know are rushing faster than you can blink to obtain the individual lashes that are sold in different lengths and colours. Dispersed flirtatiously among your real lashes, the shorter ones should be attached to the corners of your eyes and the longest ones kept for the middle. (To avoid coming to a sticky end, allow the glue to set for a few moments before applying the lashes.) To conceal your deception, apply a smoky line of colour to the base of the lash line (this will help disguise the glue), and remember to curl the false ones as well as your real set.

MASCARA TIPS

1 Avoid the tendency to pump the wand up and down to give it an even coverage of mascara. This action just traps air inside the tube, and the mascara will dry out more quickly.

2 Remember that clear mascara is natural-looking, gives a slightly dewy look, works well with minimal make-up, and can also double up as a styling agent to shape the brows.

3 Apply mascara to false lashes in exactly the same way that you would to your own, taking special care not to rip them out of place with your eyelash comb.

Born of the fashion for body art and decoration, pretty eyelash jewels will make you sparkle at any party. Spread evenly across the lash line, or just dotted here and there as you please, they are one way to make sure everyone notices the twinkle in your eye.

MASCARA FUDGES

1 If your eyelashes run even thinner than your patience in the quest for the perfect supermodel sweep, invest in a thickening mascara. These usually contain silicones which beef up the appearance of your natural set and, particularly if combined with a few false lashes, will create the illusion of a generous fringing.

2 If your eyelashes are so short they simply look like stubbly regrowth, a lengthening mascara is your dream product. Its microscopic fibres will attach themselves to the ends of your natural lashes, and create the illusion of a lengthy pair of flutterers. (Avoid these mascaras if you have sensitive eyes.)

3 Lashings of waterproof mascara will see even the most sentimental wearer through tear-jerking moments without leaving you looking like Dirk Bogarde in the final scene of *Death In Venice*.

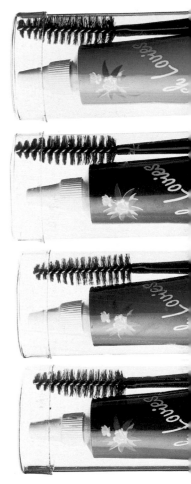

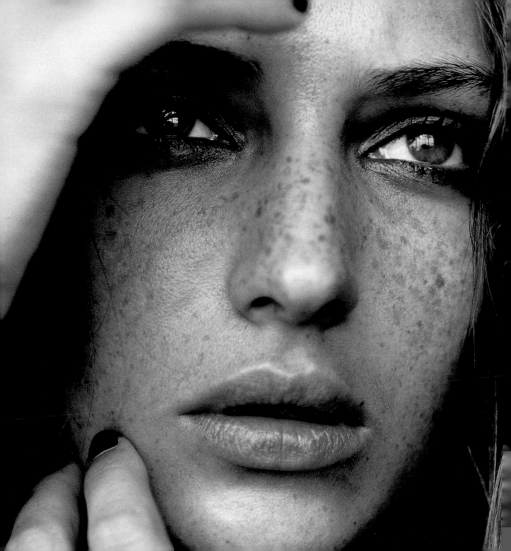

eyeshadow

Bar our mother's lipstick, eyeshadow is often the first make-up we experiment with as teenagers. This makes it all the more surprising that after years of practice, most of us are still no nearer to mastering the subtle art of blending shades than we were when we started. While a beautifully made-up eyelid looks deceptively simple to accomplish, the reality is far from easy, and achieving a sophisticated finish (as opposed to looking like we went three rounds with Tyson) is something that evades us.

Believe it or not, the trick is to keep it simple. Any make-up artist will tell you that getting it right with just one colour will enhance your look tremendously, so until you are really confident stick to single-shade application. The means is vital to the end, so chuck out the nasty sponge-tip applicator that comes with many products. A proper eyeshadow brush is worth the investment (see Tools of the Trade, page 107) – it will help the shadow glide on easily and ensure a finer finish.

Just a decade ago, the mere thought of applying eyeshadow was enough to send even the most confident make-up aficionado wild with despair. However, the appliance of science in recent years has taken the fear out of getting started. Today, it is not only colour that counts – the texture and skincare benefits of modern eyeshadow mean that colour glides on effortlessly and grips the lid without crumbling or creeping. Thanks to silicone-based ingredients which are now used to suspend colour pigments, the creation of 'truer', non-streak colours at both ends of the market is now possible. Texture (the buzz word of modern make-up) has seen a radical change in medium too – eyeshadows are now available in powder, gel, cream and mousse form, and these add colour to your lids while simultaneously reducing the appearance of surface lines and wrinkles. Throw out past taboos about colour, and experiment with whatever shade takes your fancy.

As the creative force behind supermarket chain Tesco's beauty range, Barbara Daly has first-hand experience in getting the most out of your eyes. 'Look what happens with young eyes,' she says. 'They look dewy and fresh and the skin around the eyes doesn't appear dry. To make your eyes look younger, try using glossy products in the corner of the eyes nearest the nose. Also use it as a highlighter on the brow bone and in the middle of the upper lid.' Remember that the lighter the shade, the more flattering the result. Ivory, cream or peachy browns, blended well, should be used from the lash line to the brow bone, and only then should a second shade be added. The simplest way to achieve a great result is to only apply the second colour from the lash line up to the crease of your eyelid. 'Mature women are best to keep away from pearlized products,' says Daly, 'as they tend to draw attention to unwanted lines and wrinkles.'

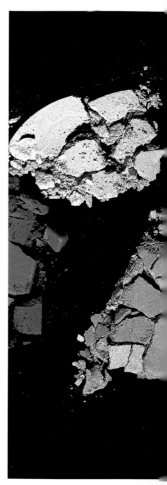

COLOUR

Fashion pundits are opting for a spectrum of bright shades, with Julien Macdonald, John Galliano and Alexander McQueen, to name but a few, sending models down the runway at their recent shows with eyes painted as brightly as their collections. If you want to add a hint of drama to your face with just a streak of one solid colour, or prefer to look like a double for *Joseph and the Amazing Technicolor Dreamcoat*, let any old-fashioned taboos fly out of the window. The point of make-up, after all, is to play and experiment. With regiments of new writers, models and make-up artists espousing rules as if each were the eleventh commandment, it is easy to forget that make-up application should be fun.

The eye is a fabulous area on which to experiment with colour. Anything from darker, depth-creating shadows to glittery, light-reflecting options and Day-Glo shades will make sure that you are the brightest spark. Although there are no hard-and-fast rules, here are a few suggestions to make your experiments more fruitful:

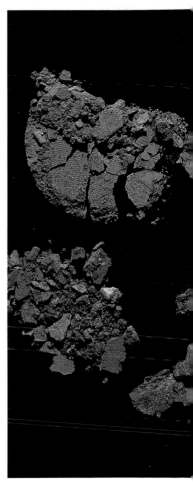

1 Colour is an excellent tool for changing your look; instead of being frightened by it, use it to your advantage. Throw out any preconceptions you have – if it feels right, wear it. The best way to ease yourself into using colour is to start by using muted tones.

2 Make sure you do not smudge your entire face with emerald green shadow by preparing properly. Apply translucent powder beneath the bottom lashes first. This will act as a magnet to any falling shadow, and can be swept away once you have finished.

3 Do not match your eyeshadow colour to your clothes or lipstick. Clashing colours always look more modern.

4 Dominique Szabo of Estée Lauder says: 'Green, yellow and brown hues are not ideal on Asian skins. Black skin is beautiful with any deep colours, like purple, red, dark blue, especially with pearlescent finishes. Fair skin looks good with browns and pastels.'

5 Always prep your eyelids with foundation or moisturizer. This will ensure eyeshadow glides on easily, and prevent the colour from cracking.

6 For those who are not a dab hand with an eyeshadow brush, cream shadows are an easy way to achieve a smooth layer of colour using your fingers. Stick to one shade if applying cream shadow.

SHADOW APPLICATION TIPS

1 Remember that just a hint of colour will change your whole look. To open up the eye area, use light or pearlized shadows, swept right up to the brow bone itself.

2 Do not use dark colours in the corner of your eyelids nearest your nose, as this will pull the eyes in, and make even the smallest nose look larger.

3 If you want a hint of colour, but do not feel like hitting the streets with fuchsia eyelids, try blue or green eyeliner pencil smudged gently around the lash line or a coloured mascara. This will give the feeling of colour in a more subtle application.

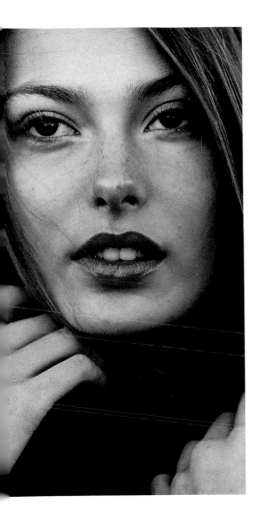

EYELINER APPLICATION TIPS

1 Eyeliner pencils give a softer effect than liquids, but best of all is a dark powder shadow line, created by using the tiniest, most pointed brush. The shadow is much subtler and gives you a sexy, doe-eyed look. Liquid liners are best left to the professionals, but if you must, use a magnifying mirror, pull the eyelid taut and apply the liner in one continuous movement as close to the lashes as possible.

2 If you're too busy to apply eyeliner daily, you could have a line permanently tattooed around the lash line. This involves injecting tiny coloured particles of iron oxide into the skin. The eye area is very delicate, so finding an experienced beauty therapist is essential. Don't let associations with other types of tattooing put you off – under-eye tattooing can look very natural. Be warned: it is usually very painful. Have a patch test first to check your skin will not react adversely, and use an antibiotic cream afterwards to ward off infection.

TEXTURES

TRADITIONAL POWDER SHADOW looks great in the evenings when you want a stronger look. Its modern no-crease formulation will make sure it glides on smoothly and does not flake.

CREAM SHADOW slides on like a second skin. It is brilliant if you are in a rush and just want to smooth it on with your fingertips. It complements a light-reflecting, non-matt foundation look and (in a neutral colour) results in a very natural look that is suitable for daytime wear.

GEL SHADOW provides a modern alternative to cream. Its colour pigments are suspended in a gel formulation that is quick and easy to apply with the fingertips. They generally stay put even if you have greasy skin, as the eye area always naturally tends to feel drier.

MULTIPURPOSE STICKS AND EYESHADOW CRAYONS were created by make-up artists to suit the time constraints of a modern lifestyle. These products are shaped like pencils (just draw colour directly on or below the lid and blend with fingertips) or like 'push-up' sticks, and they can be applied to cheeks and lips, as well as eyes.

ALL THAT SHIMMERS

High-sheen products have become something of a fashion staple, so it is essential to know your glitter from your gloss.

1 Pearlized shadows glide on smoothly with a brush and create a subtle shimmer, so the more mature face is able to carry them off.

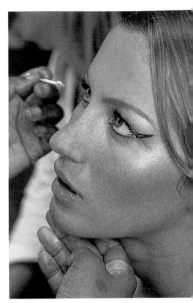

2 Shimmery creams are easier to apply than powder, as they do not disperse and leave you with glitter in unwanted places. They look like a second skin, even when applied in bright colours.

3 For a glitzy night out, a judicious amount of glitter mixed with Vaseline and applied to the eyelids will ensure you shine out.

4 White pearlized shadow acts as a superb highlighter. Sweep it up to the brow bone and line your eyes with smoky pencil, to create a wide-eyed effect. This look works very well with glossy lips, and the shadow can also be used in the centre of your mouth.

the eyes have it

NATURAL EYES

The natural eye is the simplest 'no make-up' look to achieve. All you have to do is master a few basic essentials:

1 Always use foundation or concealer to moisturize the eyelid before applying your other make-up. This creates a smooth base, and helps colour glide on smoothly.

2 Brush the eyelid very gently with a translucent powder.

3 Take one natural eyeshadow (a peach or a brownish colour) that picks up your natural skin tone, and, using a good, medium-sized brush, coat the lid, starting at the lash line and working right up towards the brow bone. Add a touch of BeneFit's High Beam to the browbone for a natural-looking highlight.

4 Next curl your eyelashes. This is a step that many women omit, but a make-up artist would never sacrifice. Creep the curler gently up the lashes, starting at the root and being sure to maintain even pressure throughout. Curled lashes open up the eye and create a deliciously sexy fan effect.

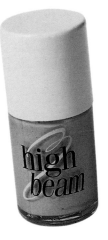

Always curl them after you have applied your eyeshadow: this will ensure you do not disturb your artfully enhanced lashes with the eyeshadow brush.

5 Apply mascara to the top lashes, concentrating on the tips. Never apply mascara directly to the roots of the lashes as it looks unnatural and creates a scary spider-leg effect.

6 If desired, apply the mascara to your lower lashes, as directed above.

7 If you prefer a 'no make-up' look, substitute transparent mascara for a coloured one.

8 Comb through your lashes with an eyelash comb before they dry.

9 Using a small eyeshadow brush (preferably either a pointed one or one with a stiff, slanted edge), line the lower lid with the same natural colour as you used before, working as close to the lash line as possible.

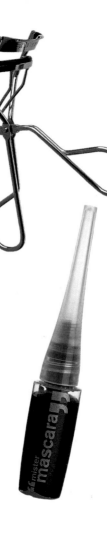

NEUTRAL EYES

These are not the same as natural eyes, as they involve more product and a cannier technique. Applied well, the neutral eye will take you from office to evening and suits everybody.

1 Apply foundation and powder to the lids.

2 Using a soft eyeshadow brush, pick up a little brown eyeshadow powder and blend it into the inner and outer corners of your eye and under the bottom lashes.

'Neutral tones can be applied in liquid, cream, shimmer or matt, each texture creating subtle differences.'

**Kevyn Aucoin
Make-up guru**

3 Next take a peachy powder shadow and gently fill in the gap left between the two brown corners. Blend well to avoid any obvious 'joining' of the products.

4 Add an ivory highlighter, starting just above the crease in the eyelid and going right up to the brow bone itself.

5 Curl the eyelashes gently with an eyelash curler, and add a coat of mascara to top and bottom lashes, sweeping outwards towards the outer edges of the eyes.

6 Comb the lashes while they are still wet, and apply a second coat before the mascara hardens.

7 Using a larger brush, dust apricot blusher along the temples and down the hairline on either side of your eyes.

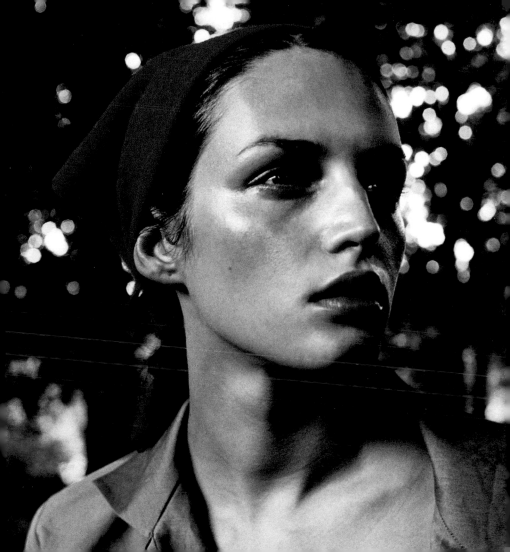

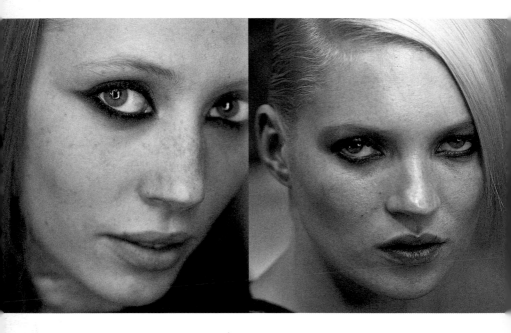

SMOKY EYES

Smoky eyes look really sultry and work best in softer, evening light.

1 First apply foundation and translucent powder to the eyelid, as in Natural Eyes on page 180.

2 Using a neutral eyeshadow, cover the whole eyelid, from the lashes right up to the brow bone.

3 Next, take a soft eyeliner pencil with a rubber hoof in black, chocolate-brown or charcoal-grey. Apply it in small, even strokes along the upper and lower lash lines, then smudge gently with the rubber tip (do not smudge with your fingers).

4 Using a dark grey eyeshadow (if you have light eyes) or a brown one (if your eyes are dark), brush colour into the crease of the eyelid, but do not go above the crease line that is created when the eye is open.

5 Curl the lashes and apply mascara, as in Natural Eyes on pages 180-1.

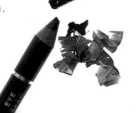

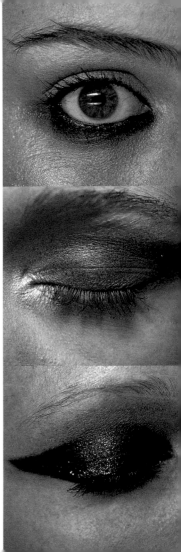

GLOSSY EYES

First used in black-and-white Hollywood films, the glossy eye has been firmly reinstated at the forefront of fashion. It looks great but requires major upkeep, so it is a definite 'no no' for everyday wear.

1 Prepare eyelids with foundation and powder as in previous looks.

2 Add a generous scoop of loose powder underneath your lower lashes. This will catch any falling colour pigments and can be swept off easily afterwards.

3 Choose your favourite single eyeshadow colour (anything from baby pink to citrus orange) and sweep it generously, and evenly, from the lash line right up to the brow bone. Gently dust off any fallen colour shadow with a large powder brush.

4 Curl your eyelashes and apply mascara at this point. Once the gloss is applied, you will run the risk of smudging your lids and eyelashes.

5 Next, cover the coloured lid with a thin coat of Vaseline, very carefully and evenly, using a brush.

6 If you want a glossy effect but can compromise on wet-look sheen in return for a look that will last a little longer, substitute Vaseline with shimmer shadow.

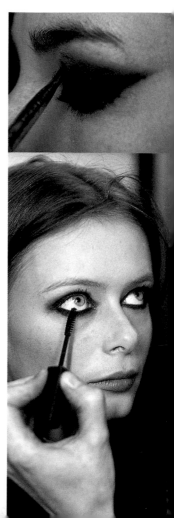

7 To complement a healthy suntan, drop the shadow altogether. Instead, apply mascara to your lashes, then coat the eyelids in Vaseline or Calvin Klein's Eye Gloss.

8 Remember that this look works best on the very young. For anyone over 35, creamy shadows are far more flattering.

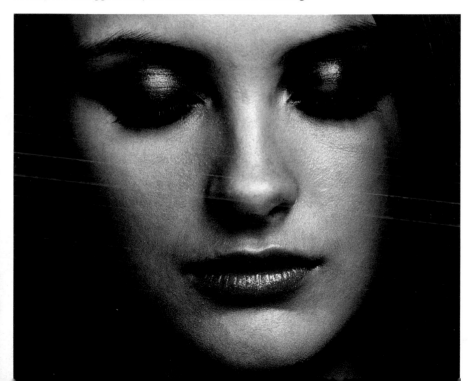

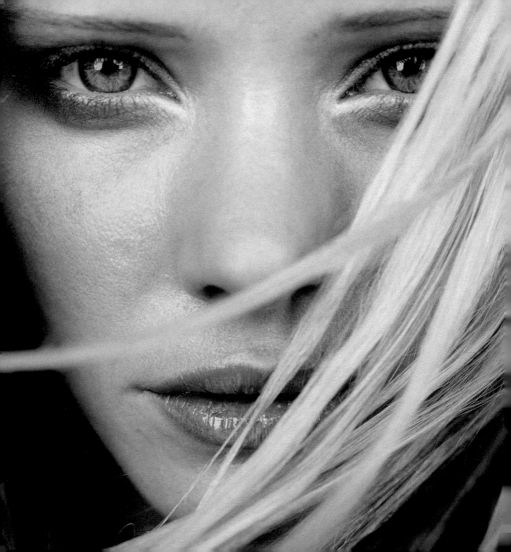

SHIMMERY EYES

Iridescent or metallic eye make-up is a brilliant complement to today's dewy or light-reflecting foundations.

1 Prepare eyelids with foundation and powder.

2 Take a warm-toned, chocolate-brown eye pencil and draw a line as close to your upper lashes as possible. Smudge this in well with an eyeshadow brush or the rubber-hoofed tip of the pencil.

3 Apply a cream shadow in a different colour (burgundy, forest green and gold all work well for this look). Apply it around the entire eye area, without covering the darkest part of the brown eyeliner (at the lash line). Blend outwards using a clean eyeshadow brush.

4 Next take a shimmery ivory powder shadow or highlighter and brush it above the coloured eye area, sweeping right up to the brow bone.

5 Lastly, apply your mascara. A coloured wand can be very effective here, as long as it is a similar tone to the coloured shadow.

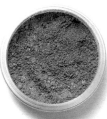

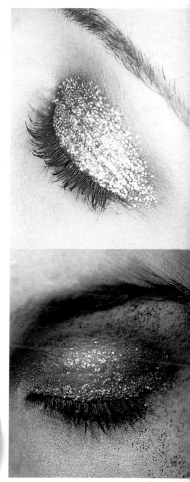

COLOURFUL EYES

Coloured eyeshadow is no longer the domain of one's grandmother. Dip in and have fun, but remember careful editing is key to carrying this look off with style.

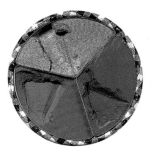

1 Prepare eyelids as always.

2 Dab plenty of loose powder underneath the eyes, to catch any falling colour pigments.

3 Take a coloured eye pencil and line the inner rim (top and bottom) of the eye.

4 Next take a liquid metallic eyeshadow two shades lighter than the pencil, and wash it over the eyelid and underneath the lower lashes with an eyebrow brush, making sure it is well blended and fades out towards the outer edges.

5 Use gold (to complement warm colour shadow) or silver (to complement cool colour shadow) liquid shadow. Apply to the centre of the upper eyelid, blending well at the edges so there is no obvious demarcation where the metallic meets the principal colour on the eyelid.

6 Curl your lashes, then apply mascara – black will give a contrasting look, while coloured mascara means a softer finish.

7 Sweep away any rogue colour with a large powder brush.

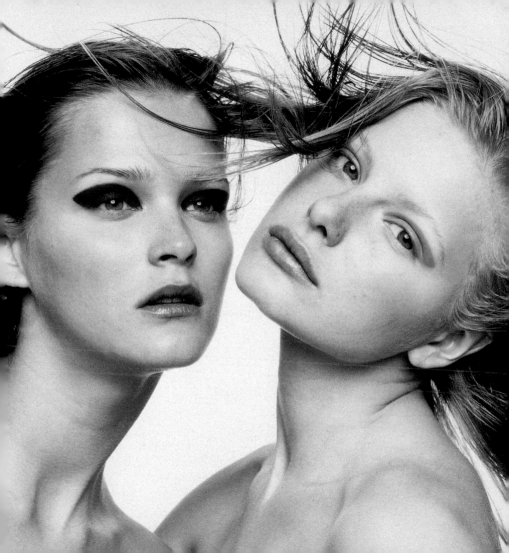

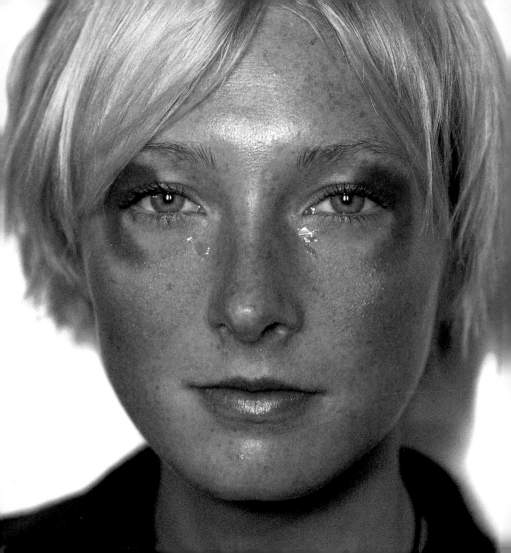

optical illusions

LIFTING 'DROOPY' EYES
Using a pencil or (if you have a very steady hand) liquid liner, draw a line along the upper lashes, extending slightly further than the corner, and sloping slightly upwards. Line the bottom lid with a colour several shades lighter than the one used on the upper lid, as this will add to the 'lift'. Then add a couple of false lashes to the outer corners of your eyes, and curl these with your natural lashes before applying mascara.

LOOKING 'BRIGHT EYED'
Create the illusion of very bright eyes by drawing inside the rim of both top and bottom lids with a white eye pencil.

INSTANT EYE JOB
Ever wondered how models always have such firm skin around their eyes? Some are born lucky, but, for others, the professional make-up artist often tapes the skin taut behind their hairline to achieve a great look for photographs. Only use this trick for the camera – you do not want the tape coming unstuck in public.

'COME TO BED' EYES

Cover the upper lids with frosted white shadow, then, in one continuous sweep, draw black eyeliner along the upper lash line, as close to the upper lashes as possible and sloping downwards. Then apply false lashes on top of your own, and push them downwards while they are drying to create a sexy, sleepy look.

MAKE-UP ARTISTS' TOP TIPS

'I don't think that women should worry too much about the shape of their eyes – I don't think that there is a 'perfect shape' anyway. Make the most of what is naturally yours, and remember that smiling eyes are by far the prettiest.'
BARBARA DALY

'Apply eye pencils at the root of the lashes, not above or under.'
LAURA MERCIER

'When lining the inner rim of the eyes, be sure the pencil tip has been blended down a bit. Avoid a very sharp point, for obvious reasons.'
KEVYN AUCOIN

'Dot under-eye concealer in very small points around the socket bone. Use a small brush to avoid overapplication, and then pat in gently with your fingertips.'
MAGGIE HUNT

'To define your eyebrows, use a light feathery action, whether you are using pencil or powder. Powder should be applied with an eyeliner brush, following the direction in which the hairs grow.'
MARY GREENWELL

CHANGING YOUR FACE SHAPE

- Conjure the illusion of a narrower jaw line by extending your eyebrows outwards, towards your hairline.

- Draw attention away from 'life jacket' lips by playing up your eyes.

- To create the illusion of a narrower nose, use a matt bronzer as a shader down the outside edges of the nose. Then use a shimmery ivory powder as a highlighter down the bridge of the nose. Only do this at night-time, as broad daylight will give the game away.

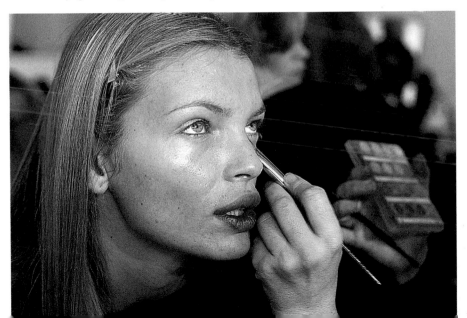

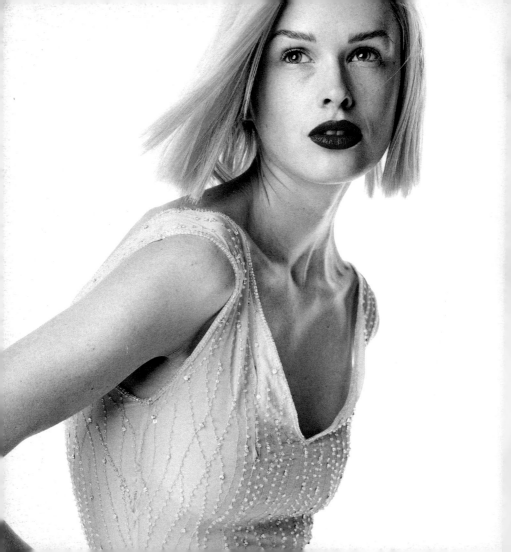

5

lips

'Dark colours tend to make lips
look smaller, but a light colour
will maximize the size of the mouth.'
Tom Pecheux, make-up artist

While most fashions go out as quickly as they come in, the trend for oversized kissers just keeps getting bigger. With the likes of Liz Hurley, Esther Candidas, Julia Roberts and Angelina Jolie as modern-day beauty icons, it is not surprising that in the past few years every girl worth her BeneFit Lip Plump has contemplated having collagen injections.

In an area where technology knows no bounds, lip moisturizers, plumpers, anti-run agents and sun protection factors are all standard features of today's products. Once nothing more than a stick of wax and pigment (which stuck to your coffee cup or your boyfriend's shirt collar), lipstick is no longer simply about colour. Like so many other make-up products, the modern lipstick is multitextured and multifunctional. And as your mouth is the most titillating area of your face, looking after it is paramount to keeping you attractive.

'Colour suitability and selection are as personal as diet: just as we choose what nutrition we ingest, we ultimately choose what make-up will express about our inner selves, in its application and styling method upon our external canvas.'

David Horne, make-up artist

PUT YOUR MONEY WHERE YOUR MOUTH IS

Considering the muscles in the mouth area are used substantially more than most of our other muscles (every time we speak, eat or smile) it is not surprising that this is also an area prone to showing giveaway signs of ageing, such as fine lines and wrinkles. The delicate skin that covers lips quickly falls prey to such external aggressors as changing weather conditions and central heating. So how do we maintain a perfect pout?

1 Whenever you expose yourself to extreme temperatures (outside cold, indoor heat or vice versa), or you are feeling slightly under the weather, the lips are liable to dehydrate and flake. Resist temptation and never nibble at bits of peeling skin.

2 Use a gentle lip exfoliator (Clinique's and Chanel's are both wonderful) that encourages desquamation (the natural shedding of cells) without harming the delicate skin that covers your lips. Do not use abrasive products here, as you will end up with a sore, scabby mouth.

3 Moisturize, moisturize, moisturize. Remember that the lips do not excrete sebum, so rely largely on topical applications to keep them tender. Licking your lips will only make them drier.

4 Look out for petroleum-based moisturizers – these seal moisture in, and keep external aggressors out. Vaseline and Elizabeth Arden's Eight Hour Cream work wonders on dry lips.

5 Always use a product with sun protection on and around the mouth. Harmful UV rays cause lips to tan (unattractive), burn (unhealthy) and age (unwanted vertical lines around the mouth).

6 To give your lips a real boost, use an intensive moisturizer at night. Your mouth is less mobile while you sleep, and because you lick off less product, it has a better chance to do some vital repair work. Intensive skin creams will often work wonders on lips, too, so you need not confine yourself to Carmex.

technology

Lipstick is possibly the oldest item of decorative cosmetic. Traditionally used simply to enhance the appearance of the user, colour was always the main focus when creating a new line. Not any more – the technological advances in skincare are carried generously into colour cosmetics as well, so the demanding consumer can now reap more from her investment. Look out for:

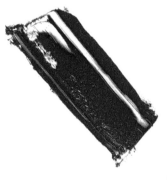

NON-TRANSFER LIPSTICKS release their colour slowly over a prolonged period of time, and thus fix the initial application of colour in place for hours on end. The only drawback is getting them off your lips at the end of the day, which entails dousing your mouth with the cosmetic equivalent of turpentine.

PRODUCTS CONTAINING WATER MOLECULES, which keep the lips moist throughout the course of the day. Remember that the skin on the lips is thinner than elsewhere on the face and very sensitive; it can quickly become dehydrated because it does not produce sebum.

DRY LIPOSOMES are ingredients which are activated by saliva and can hold water for hours. Mixed with colour pigments, they make an ideal moisturizer for the lips.

ANTIOXIDANT VITAMINS A AND E are routinely included in today's lipsticks to guard against the free-radical damage that would otherwise lead to premature ageing of the skin around the mouth.

SUN PROTECTION FACTORS are essential ingredients for protecting the delicate skin of the lips against damage caused by invasive ultraviolet rays. Suntanned lips are unattractive, in any case.

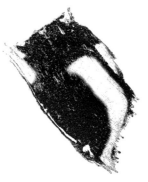

LIP FACTS

1 97 per cent of women aged between 20 and 35 wear lipstick.
2 60 per cent of women own more than ten lipsticks.
3 Kylie Minogue uses Estée Lauder Pure Color Crystal Lipstick.
4 Brooke Shields uses Burt's Beeswax Lip Balm.

feathering

Unsightly feathering around the lips is often a hereditary trait, but smoking and exposure to the sun are the two main external factors that are most responsible for exacerbating the problem. Loss of skin firmness, which comes with the depletion of the skin's elastic collagen and elastin fibres, leads to the formation of characteristic vertical lines around the mouth. These are impossible to camouflage with make-up, and cause lipstick to 'bleed', which results in a messy, ungroomed and sadly aged appearance.

'Permanent pleats are very nice for skirts and trousers, but the last place you want them is around the mouth,' says Dr Daniel Maes, the vice president of Research and Development for Estée Lauder Worldwide. 'Unfortunately, however, this particularly vulnerable area loses its ability to resist the signs of stress quite easily, and the vertical lines that form here may be even more pronounced than the lines anywhere else on the face.'

natural born fillers

When it comes to lips, we do not have to age glaringly or indeed, age much at all. Though we cannot hold on to our own collagen and elastin fibres for ever, we can re-create the firm and youthful texture that we lose as we get older by 'filling' our lips with a variety of treatments. European cosmetic surgeons are at the forefront of 'filler' technology, with new alternatives being tested almost every month. However, all cosmetic procedures carry an element of risk, so be sure to find a reputable practitioner (recommended by a doctor or someone else who has consulted him or her) before undergoing treatment.

COLLAGEN

Collagen is still the most widely used and known lip enlarger, and its use for more than two decades makes it the most tried and tested way to inflate your lips to date. Derived from the collagen that is naturally present in cow hides, it is available in three forms: Zyderm, Zyplast and Resoplast. Injected into the lips, it increases the size of your pouters for up to three months or even more. The downside of collagen injections is that they can cause allergic reactions in some people, so it is important that a small patch test be carried out before treatment commences.

ALLODERM AND DERMOLOGEN

Processed from the skin of human corpses, Alloderm and Dermologen are used to create lips of which Hannibal Lector would be proud. Alloderm is introduced as an implant that is threaded through the lips under local anaesthetic; Dermologen is injected rather like collagen. The upside of choosing these unsavoury-sounding treatments is that allergic reactions are rare. Alloderm is a permanent treatment, but Dermologen has to be repeated after about six months, and can be painful.

ISOLOGEN AND AUTOLOGEN

For those who do not have a taste for human cadavers, these two products provide a more palatable alternative. Autologen and Isologen are forms of collagen removed from your own skin, which eliminates the chance of rejection or allergic reaction.

AUTOLOGOUS FAT TRANSPLANTATION

This treatment involves the transfer of fat taken from your own body (usually around the buttock area) to your lips. The fat is removed, curled up and slid through a tunnel hollowed out of the upper lip. It can leave a scar at the site where the graft was taken, but it causes no adverse reactions and is reabsorbed by the body after about a year.

RESTYLANE AND HYLAFORM GEL

Good alternatives for those who are allergic to collagen, these gels have the same chemical structure as enzymes that are found naturally in the skin, so they do not usually cause adverse reactions. The results last for about a year.

GORE-TEX

Until recently Gore-Tex was most familiar from its employment in weatherproof hiking gear. Now also used by cosmetic surgeons, Gore-Tex is threaded through the lip line. It can often be felt by the patient well after treatment though reportedly not by anybody kissing them. Because the strip of Gore-Tex gradually becomes surrounded by scar tissue, it can plump up the lips by as much as 60 per cent. Downsides are similar to those of silicone: if infection sets in, the Gore-Tex has to be cut out, which can be disfiguring and distressing.

BOTOX

This is an injectable filler derived from botulinum toxin A, which causes food poisoning; it is controversially used to fill in the grooves that can run from your mouth to your nose. Some cosmetic surgeons believe it should not be used on this part of the face because it works by paralysing muscles, and is too risky to play around with. Botox injections need to be repeated every six months or so, but in some cases eventually do not need repeating because the muscle being paralysed eventually 'forgets' the way it used to move around, and thus stops forming wrinkles.

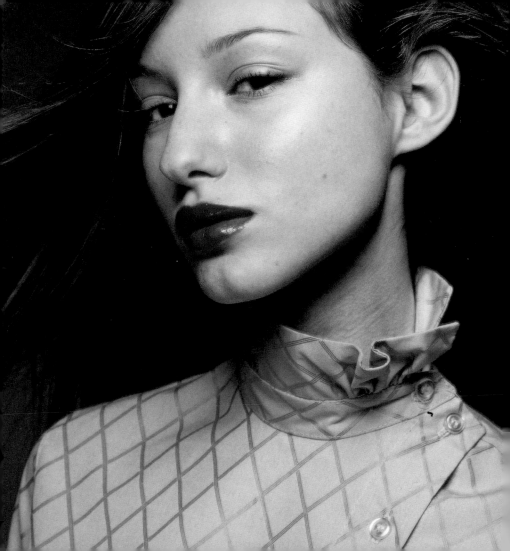

lipsticks

COLOUR

Skin tone is and is not important when it comes to choosing lipstick, but for those who think making bold statements with their lip colour is best left to those with more pout than clout, a classic look is the safest option. With a galaxy of shades and tones available, the simplest way to choose exactly the right shade for you is to stick within the colour chart traditionally associated with your skin tone. Of course, today's beauty mantra is that anyone can wear any colour, but for classicists some simple rules apply. The English rose with pink-toned skin is always best suited to 'cooler' colours (look for blue reds, blue oranges and blue pinks), while darker, Mediterranean types and those with Asian skins will enhance their features with orange-based shades. No colour is out of bounds, but if you want to play by the (traditional) rules, there will be a right red and a wrong red, a right pink and a wrong pink for you. Black skins have the greatest choice of all – a whole spectrum of colours from the palest pastel to the boldest brights look great on dark complexions. Lastly, remember that hair colour is irrelevant to lipstick choice – Snow White and Pocahontas might both sport raven locks, but their skin tone (and hence their choice of lipstick) are absolutely worlds apart.

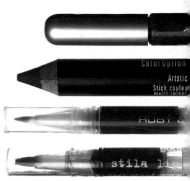

TEXTURES

LIP GLOSSES

Slick and sexy, and super for moisturizing the lips, glosses come in every variety from low sheen to high gloss. Wear with lip pencil, on its own or over a matt lipstick for a lighter effect. Lip gloss looks great, but transfers easily, can feel 'jammy' and is not long-lasting.

LIP STAINS

These do just that. For those who prefer minimal coverage these lipsticks leave the wearer with a hint of colour, rather like the look your mouth has when you have just been eating berries.

CREAMY LIPSTICKS

Smooth, youthful and suitable for all ages, these usually contain silicones to help them glide on easily.

MATT LIPSTICKS

These are long-lasting, as they do not slide around like creamy colours. However, a matt lipstick can be drying and can accentuate lines in older lips. Be sure to moisturize your lips if this is your lipstick choice, and be aware that matt lipsticks make the lips look smaller.

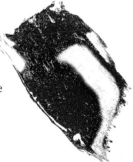

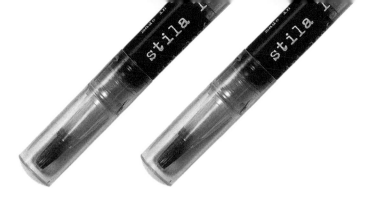

LONG-LASTING LIPSTICKS

These will stay the course as long as you do, but will have to be removed with the cosmetic equivalent of paint stripper.

SHEER LIPSTICKS

Ultra-light lipsticks, which usually have a slight sheen – these will not rub off as quickly as traditional lip gloss.

SHIMMERY LIPSTICKS

Frosted colours look fabulous, but can be ageing on anyone over 35. Their light-reflecting properties create a fuller, moist appearance.

LIP PALETTES

Long used by make-up artists, lip palettes enable you to create your own spectrum of lip shades (or draw upon a brand's ready-made selection). Laura Mercier and Bobbi Brown do the ultimate compacts.

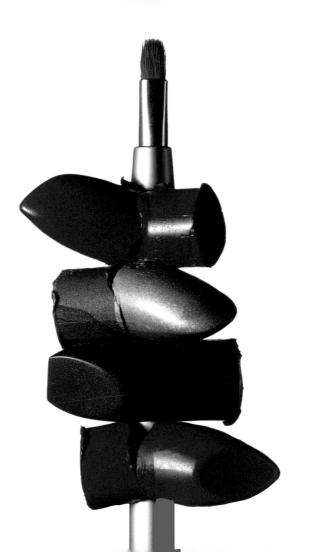

application techniques

1 Always use a brush when applying lipstick. This gives you more control over the product, and allows you to get right into the corners without smudging. It also ensures you keep your colour within your lip line and not smudged over the edges.

2 When applying lip liner, make sure your lip pencil is not too sharp to avoid creating a harsh outline. Use it very lightly to trace the outer edges of your lips, and keep your lips relaxed to avoid creating unnatural shapes.

3 Thanks to technological advances, we can now pump up our volume (to a certain extent) without having to resort to drastic measures such as cosmetic surgery. BeneFit's Lip Plump and similar wands promise to give you voluptuous lips within seconds of application.

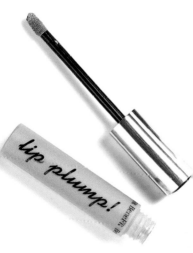

4 When using clear gloss over a coloured lipstick, first apply the gloss to your wrist, and then transfer it to your lips with a separate lip brush. Avoid using the sponge-tip applicator that comes with the gloss because it will become discoloured.

5 Wash your lip brushes regularly using a mild detergent to prevent your lip shades blending.

MAKE-UP ARTISTS' TOP TIPS

'I use pencil all over the lips, and then apply face powder on top to set the pencil. Next I apply gloss or lipstick on top. In selecting a lip pencil do not be afraid to choose a colour that is different from your lipstick. Provided the pencil is used all over the lip, applying different colours on top can create winning combinations. The notion of having to use a matching pencil and lipstick is totally old-fashioned.'
FRANÇOIS NARS

'I prefer to use a lip brush when filling in the mouth (it gives me more control than using the container), and I like to "sample" my lipsticks in a box (by colours). I actually break them off, and smudge them in. In this way they appear more like an artist's palette.'
KEVYN AUCOIN

'To create a pouty look use a pinky-brown lipstick all over the lips, and then dab a bit of concealer in the middle of the bottom lip.'
JEANINE LOBELL OF STILA COSMETICS

'Apply Vaseline and then buff with a baby's toothbrush to get rid of dry skin if you suffer from dry lips.'
BARBARA DALY

'Lip liner defines the mouth and makes lipstick last longer. On black skins I sometimes use brown eye pencil as a lip liner.'
MARY GREENWELL

'Always apply a good lip balm, and allow it to be absorbed thoroughly before you apply your lipstick. If your lips are very dry, or still moist from the balm, your lipstick won't stay put for long. Build up depth by applying lipstick, then blotting with a tissue to create a stain. Finish with a final coat for a long-lasting result.'
BOBBI BROWN

'To avoid embarrassing lipstick stains on your teeth, pop a finger inside your mouth, gently shut your lips, and pull your finger out.'
MAGGIE HUNT

FOR LONGER-LASTING LIPS

1 Always blot your lipstick with a tissue and then reapply to build up colour and durability.

2 Always apply foundation (and, if you wish, a whisper of translucent powder) to the lips before you start applying lipstick. This will prevent naturally high-coloured lips from sabotaging your desired lip colour, minimize feathering and also ensure that your lipstick stays put for longer.

3 Using a blunt lip pencil, colour in the whole lip area before you apply your lipstick over the top. This will create a stain that will last for the whole evening. Either use a pencil that matches your lipstick to maintain its true colour, or experiment by using different coloured pencils under your lipstick to create different shades.

4 Choose matt lipsticks, which last longer than glosses.

5 If you are wearing lip gloss, only apply it at the last minute to prolong its life span.

SALAD DAYS

Change your lipstick with the times if you do not want to look like a throwback. Here are some habits to avoid:

1 Lining the outline of your lips with a dark colour, and filling them in with a totally different shade.

2 Creating 'points' with your lip liner around the cupid's bow.

3 Applying lipstick blind, so that your upper lip looks like one continuous line with no cupid's bow at all.

4 Wearing a lip colour to match your outfit.

5 Wearing pearlized lipsticks if you have passed the 40 milestone (and that is being generous) – leave them for the youthful and move on to something more sophisticated.

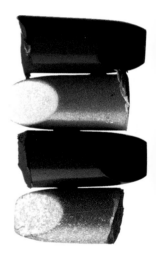

lip liners

The secret weapon in your armoury, the lip liner, used masterfully, is the quickest means of changing your lip shape. Used wrongly, or with a heavy hand, it will leave you looking more Ugly Sister than Cinderella.

While no make-up artist would be without a lip liner, the majority of women are rather scared of a product that most wrongly associate with looking unnatural and out of date. Produced in a multitude of colours and consistencies (anything from matt to pearlized to creamy), today's lip liners blend beautifully with the natural tone and texture of the skin. Available in traditional pencil, push-up crayon and felt-tip form, they are simple to use and easy to carry.

For a modern look, always run the pencil over the back of your hand after sharpening before you actually line your lips. This will soften a very pointed tip, and ensure a more natural-looking outline. Always fill in the whole lip area with the same lip liner, otherwise when your lipstick fades you will be left with an obvious outline. A peachy lip liner used like this makes a great alternative to lipstick for a daytime look.

If the lip liner you are using is too dark, tone it down with a little foundation. Keep your lips relaxed, and do not press too hard when applying lip liner. Using small feathery movements will keep the line looking more natural, but be careful not to end up with a broken lip line.

SEMI-PERMANENT MAKE-UP

If you cannot be bothered to line your lips every time you go out, but like the effect that is achieved when you have done it, semi-permanent make-up (or a tattooed lip line) may be the answer for you. Many a celebrity who has decided against collagen has opted to enhance her pout with a subtle tattoo – very effective, and far less obvious. The process involves injecting colour pigments around the shape of your natural lip line, in a shade that blends imperceptibly with your lips. The upsides to this are that it is low maintenance, and you will leave home every day with a pair of perfectly defined lips. The downsides are that it can be painful, some people have had allergic reactions, and it does not last for ever (treatments need to be repeated on average every three months). If you do choose to take this route, make sure that you find a reputable therapist, because ensuing infections can be nasty.

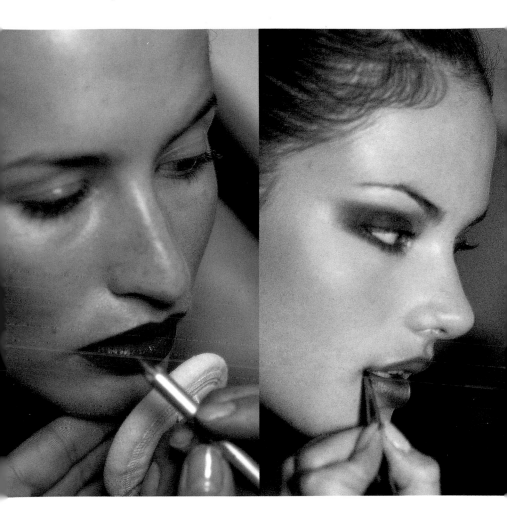

CREATING DIFFERENT LIP SHAPES

Change your lip shape, and at once you send out different messages about yourself. If you were not born with lips big enough to rival Mick Jagger's (or were, but do not like them) a little cosmetic artistry can go a long way to improve what nature gave you.

OBSERVE THE GROUND RULES

Before you apply any colour, make sure your base is properly applied. Lips should be covered in foundation or concealer, and brushed with a whisper of translucent powder, to disguise your natural lip line and to create a 'fixer' for the new lip shape that you are about to apply.

NATURAL LIPS

If you are content with your lip shape, take a sharp lip liner, and run it against the back of your hand. Then relax the mouth and gently trace your natural lip shape with the pencil. Fill in the lips, lightly, with the same pencil, and finally coat with clear gloss to finish the look.

TO CREATE A FULLER MOUTH

1 Using a slightly blunter lip liner, trace outside your upper lip line, following its natural shape and ensuring that the edge of the lip liner is still touching your natural lip line. (This is very important, because if the liner does not touch your natural lip line, you could be left with a giveaway gap if your lipstick budges.) Check that you like the shape you have achieved, and then follow the same principle for the bottom lip. If you make a mistake, remove the line with cleanser on a cotton bud (Q-Tip), and then reapply concealer to the exposed area before starting again.

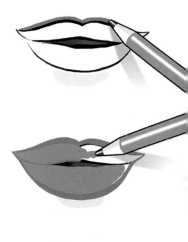

2 Fill in the new lip area with the pencil, using very light pressure, so that the outline still looks darker than the inside.

3 Then, take a lip gloss and paint over the whole mouth area using a lip brush.

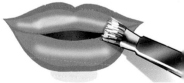

4 Add a sliver of silver as a highlighter to the centre of the bottom lip for added fullness (bottom). Remember that light, glossy colours create the appearance of a fuller lip, so avoid anything too dark or too matt.

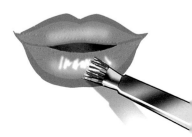

TO CREATE A THINNER MOUTH

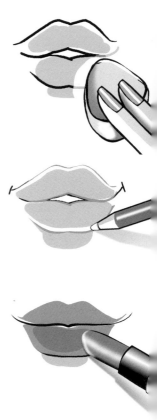

1 Use foundation on your lips to provide a base, even out any discoloration, and work as a fixative for lipstick.

2 Trace just inside your lip line with a natural-coloured pencil. Even if your chosen lip colour is different, the look will be more natural if you use a neutral liner.

3 For filling in, choose a matt colour, which absorbs light instead of reflecting it, helping to make the mouth appear smaller. Either opt for the 'dark slash' look, or detract attention from the mouth by filling in the new lip shape with a neutral liner, and creating dramatic eyes, instead.

the shape of lips to come

When it comes to cosmetic enhancement, there is nothing like a slick of your favourite lipstick. Whatever your lip shape, there are a few tricks which will guarantee that you'll know how to get mouthy when you need to.

LOOKING AS IF YOU HAVEN'T TRIED

1 Apply foundation to the lips as always.

2 Follow your natural lip shape with a neutral lip liner that picks up your skin tone. MAC's Spice is many a supermodel's favourite, and suits most people.

3 Fill in the lip shape with the lip liner, then take a swab of cotton wool and dab it over the lips for a softening effect.

4 Using your fingertip, apply a spot of clear gloss to the centre of your bottom lip, and smack your lips together.

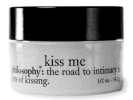

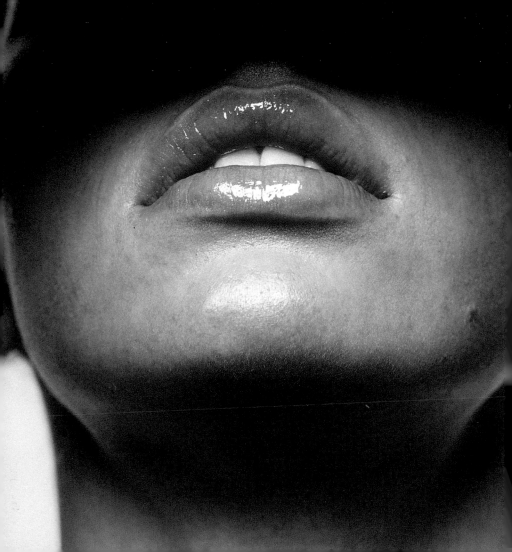

HERE COMES THE BRIDE

1 Cover the lips well with foundation.

2 Outline your natural lip shape using a pinkish pencil. Remember that your wedding is not a fancy dress party – you should look like the best possible version of yourself, and avoid the temptation to create an alter ego who you will not recognize in your wedding photographs.

3 Fill in the lips with the lip pencil, blot with a tissue, and then fill in again. This is the best way to ensure that your lip colour lasts all day, and not just for the ceremony and photographs.

4 Choose a creamy lipstick (in a pinkish-brown tone) over any other texture. Matt lipstick is too harsh for a bride, gloss is too tacky and a stain too minimal. Using a good lip brush, fill in the lip shape, taking great care not to smudge lipstick outside the lip line.

5 Blot lips with a tissue, and reapply.

6 It truly is best to stick to natural tones on your wedding day – nothing looks worse than a bride, delicately decked out in ivory, walking down the aisle with a pair of crimson kissers.

GLOSSY LIPS

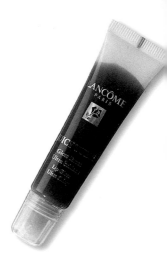

1 Gently buff your lips with a baby's toothbrush, or a lip exfoliating cream.

2 This is the only look where you don't need to cover lips in foundation. (If you do, your mouth will look too pale.)

3 Line lips with a blunt lip liner, and smudge to prevent a line of demarcation.

4 Use a lip brush to fill in lips with a high-sheen gloss. Avoid roll-ons as they are hard to control and could smudge.

5 Only apply one coat of lip gloss, to maintain a clean, reflective look.

6 If you want to add colour, apply a matt lipstick, blot, reapply and then top with clear lip gloss. Don't put a lip brush with coloured lipstick into a lip gloss container as the pigment is impossible to remove.

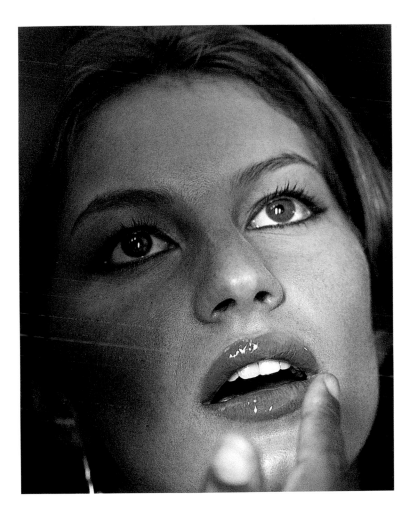

THE ROSEBUD MOUTH

1 Apply a little foundation or concealer to the sides of the lips and blend it in well so that the outside of your mouth 'disappears' into your foundation.

2 Using a dark lip liner, and starting inside the edges of your natural mouth, draw a new upper lip line that is generously rounded around the cupid's bow. Then, again starting inside the edge of your natural lower lip, trace a new line with a gentle fullness in the middle.

3 Fill in the new lip shape with your lip liner, making sure that the corners of the mouth turn up slightly.

4 Using a creamy lipstick, in a similar shade to the lip liner, cover the lips, blot with a tissue, and reapply.

5 This lip shape is usually 'bleed free', which makes it a good one for when you are wearing darker colours, of which the high pigment concentration often causes them to wander unflatteringly.

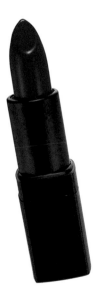

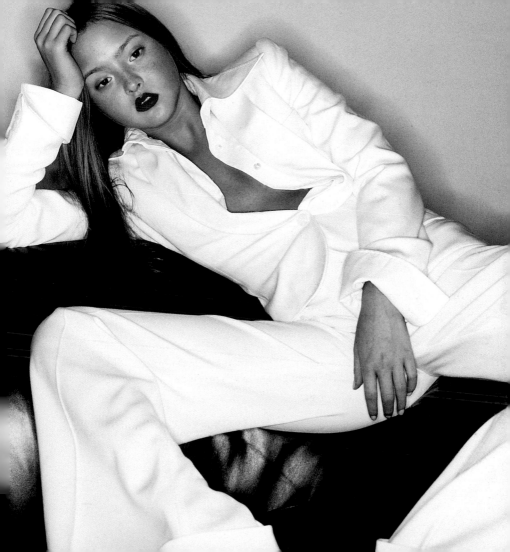

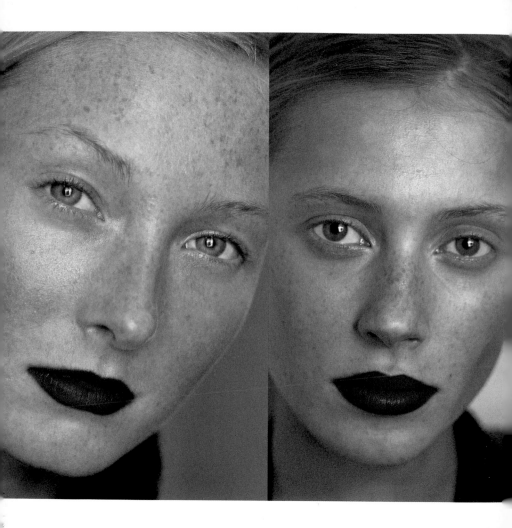

CLASSIC RED

1 Prepare the lips with a good base as always.

2 Follow your own lip shape with a neutral lip liner, in a colour that blends with your natural skin tone. At the cupid's bow, so as not to exaggerate the 'points', relax your mouth and ensure that your pencil is not too sharp. Fill in the mouth with the same colour.

3 Next take a creamy red lipstick (with blue tones if you have pink-toned skin, or orange tones if you have yellow-toned skin) and fill in the mouth.

4 Blot with a tissue and reapply.

5 For a classic finish, avoid matt lipsticks (two-dimensional) and glosses (too Hollywood). Never use red lip pencil with red lipstick, as it looks unnatural.

RED

Red is the one colour that crosses the generations – a timeless classic that bridges the gaps of age and culture. Ultimately vampish and always sexy, a pair of red lips has emblazoned icons such as Marilyn Monroe, Paloma Picasso and Eva Perón on our memories for ever.

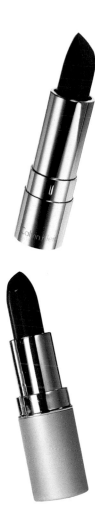

MATT LIPS

1 Thoroughly moisturize lips before applying foundation. Then line in a lip liner close to your natural colour for a hip, up-to-the-minute look.

2 Next, using a matt lipstick of your choice, fill in the lip area with a lip brush. Blot and reapply.

3 Add a touch of colour one shade lighter than your chosen lipstick to the centre of both top and bottom lips to stop the look becoming completely flat.

STAINED LIPS

1 Prepare the lips as always. Although a stained look gives the impression that your lipstick has worn off, it only works if the stain itself will go the distance.

2 You can create a stained look with any of the lip shapes covered before, but as this is quite a low-maintenance look, following your natural lip line with a pencil that matches your chosen lip colour usually gives the best results. Fill in with the same pencil.

3 Using a sheer lipstick, fill in the entire mouth with colour. Deep jewel colours work best for this look, lending the lips a sensual, lickable allure. Blot and reapply.

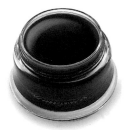

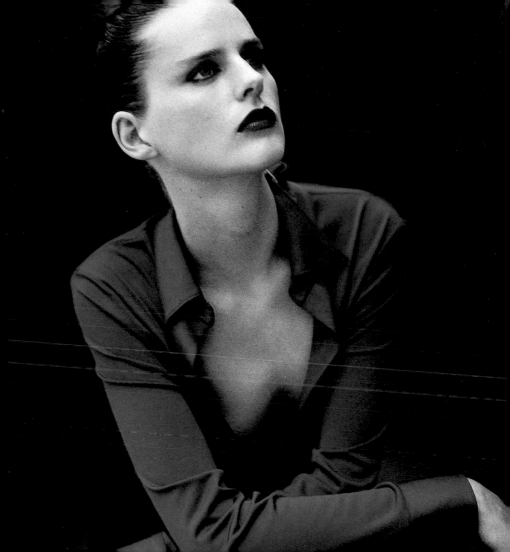

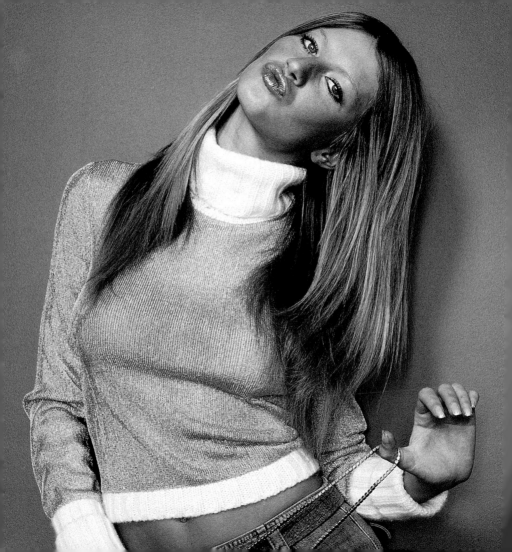

THE PARIS POUT

1 Blot out your natural lips with foundation, and finish with a whisper of translucent powder to make a smooth canvas for your new mouth.

2 Take a lip liner of your choice (this can either be neutral or match your lipstick) and, starting slightly outside your natural lip line, draw gently upwards towards the peak of the lips. Create a rounded shape that ends just above the centre of your top lip, and just below the centre of your bottom lip.

3 Then, carefully fill in the new lip shape with lip liner.

4 Using a creamy-textured lipstick that is a shade or two darker than your main lipstick colour, fill in the corners of the new mouth shape with a firm lip brush.

5 Using a clean brush, fill in the rest of the lips with lipstick in either a gloss or a pearlized finish. Blend carefully where the main colour joins the colour in the corners of the lips, taking care not to cover the deeper shade entirely.

6 Then carefully coat the lips with a layer of clear gloss.

7 Add a dab of silver lipstick to the centre of the bottom lip, and also to the cupid's bow. This will create a three-dimensional effect, and give the lips a 'cushioned' appearance.

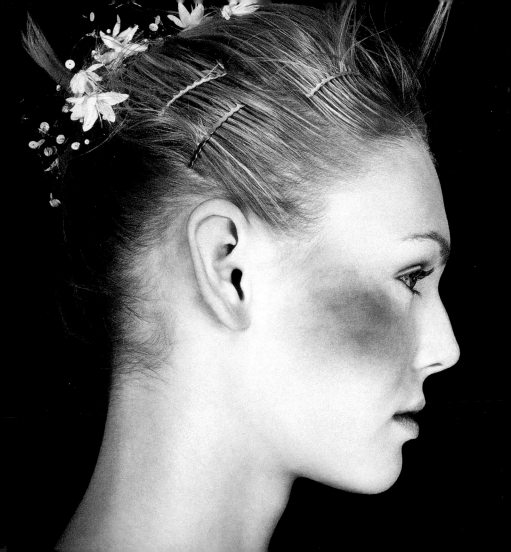

6 cheeks

'The right blusher for you is the same
colour your cheeks are naturally
when you're really healthy.'
Bobbi Brown, make-up guru

One of the make-up basics, blusher is a constant stumbling block for many women. While fashions for where to apply it come and go, getting your technique right is always vital. A little too much, the wrong shade or applied at slightly the wrong angle, and you may end up more Coco the Clown than Coco Chanel.

It is all too easy to get trapped in a 'salad days' application, but what looked fine then rarely translates successfully to today. Likewise, taking up-to-the-minute trends too literally does not work (unless, of course, you happen to look like Kate Moss or Liberty Ross). Fuchsia cheeks with startling white highlighter are best left to glossy magazine spreads, and you can wave goodbye to the liberal-handed application of 'Aunt Sally' circles, unless they are brilliantly touched in for you by a professional make-up artist. Moderation is the name of the game if you want beautiful results. Although the price of a good blusher brush can seem like bare-faced cheek, it should be viewed as a wise long-term investment. Treated well (which means washed regularly in lukewarm soapy water and then laid flat to dry), a brush by Shu Uemura, for example, should last years, and will make all the difference to your application.

The plethora of colours available today makes choice harder, but sticking to pinks and peaches works well for most women. These hues enhance natural skin tones, and are more forgiving if you are not a dab hand at application. Do not be put off by shades that look vivid in their container –

'Blush is the one piece of make-up you will never have to change. Stick with a blush that adds the right healthy glow, and you can always change the colour of your eyes or lips to alter your look.'

Mary Greenwell,
make-up artist

just a whisper, deftly applied across the apple of the cheek, often results in a fine, subtle finish. While cult brands Nars, MAC and Stila offer a superb and ever-enlarging palette of shades, I personally always keep to the traditional houses of Chanel, YSL and Christian Dior – their products' purity of colour and silky texture are pretty hard to beat.

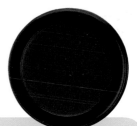

MAKE-UP ARTISTS' TOP TIPS

'I like to use two layers of blusher, with a little translucent powder sandwiched in between. I find it helps the colour stay put for longer. I also use a face shaper in a matt brown to minimize chubby cheeks and high foreheads. Choose a shade of powder that is a darker version of your own skin tone, and brush it onto heavy areas to make them recede.'
MAGGIE HUNT

'Don't just apply blusher to the cheeks. A light application of blush to the temples, forehead and chin brings the face together. I find the best way to apply powder blush is to shake or blow off any excess from your blush brush first, then sweep it across all the areas I've mentioned.'
KEVYN AUCOIN

'Blush is my favourite thing in the world; if you have the right blush you look younger, fresher, prettier. Older women should add a tawny blush (it looks more natural than corals or reds) to their list of basics. It becomes more important as you mature, because the skin cells don't turn over so quickly, and the skin doesn't look as fresh. Sometimes I use two blushers – a neutral one and then a brighter one on top. The darker your colouring, the more blush you need.'
BOBBI BROWN

textures

POWDERS

The mainstay of blusher application, powders are easy to apply and can easily be layered for a lighter or a deeper finish. Thanks to developments in today's technology, powder blushers are now available in non-crease formulations and glide on easily without going patchy. Peaches and pinks suit most people, and bestow a natural finish that looks great used sparingly in daylight or deepened for more dramatic effect at night.

LIQUID BLUSHERS

Usually packaged in a tube, liquid blushers are best applied and blended with the fingertips and give a light, natural coverage. Ideal for holidays, hot weather or when you are slightly suntanned, they supply minimal coverage to maximum effect.

CREAM BLUSHERS

Much like the traditional 'rouge', but in a far sleeker formulation, today's cream blushers are very easy to apply and do not streak. If you are not a dab hand with a brush, cream blusher is easy to control with your fingertips (but do

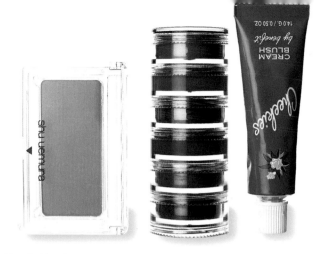

remember to blend, blend, blend to avoid the zebra effect) and it gives a more natural daytime finish than powder. It also has a youthful, light-reflecting finish. A make-up artist's trick is to apply a whisper of translucent powder on top of cream blush, which makes the colour look as if it really is coming from within. Cream blush is particularly effective for drier and more mature skins, as it will not creep into wrinkles like a powder can.

HIGHLIGHTING STICKS AND LOTIONS

These come in a variety of shades from warm to cool, and can be used all over the face or on specific areas such as cheeks or brow bones to accentuate their shape. François Nars makes the Rolls-Royce of sticks. Do not be inhibited by labelling – these sticks are multipurpose and add an alluring glow to décolletage and shoulder blades, as well as the face.

GLITTER POWDERS

Glitter powders impart a 'stardust' look and add a modern, light-reflecting quality to your appearance.

GLITTERY LIQUIDS

Easier to apply than the traditional highlighters – while giving a similar end result – these add a subtle sheen.

GELS

Colour pigments suspended in a gel formulation are among the newest types of blusher to hit the market. Excellent for oily skins, they slip less than cream products, as the gel dries out to leave the faintest whisper of colour over the cheek. The most transparent form of cheek colour, gel blushers are superb for summer. They should always be applied directly over moisturizer or foundation to help them glide on more easily. Wash your hands after application, to avoid the pigment staining.

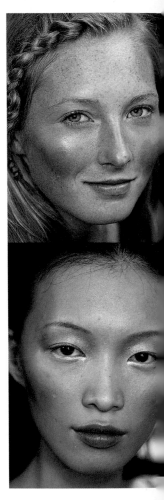

colour matching

Cheek colour should always be used to add life and vitality to your complexion, rather than to change your natural skin tone. There is no greater beauty error than trying to counteract a vivid complexion with a dull cheek shade. If you do suffer from high coloration, tone it down with a primer (see page 80), then use a pink- or peach-toned blusher to bring back a natural-looking glow. Those with dark skins should avoid 'blue'-toned shades (usually found in the pink family) and opt for warmer ones such as apricot and orange. Anything from the sheerest whisper to a bold and striking colour statement looks great on darker skins, but Asians and English roses are best advised to stick to a subtler approach in order to prevent looking like a rag doll with big discs of colour painted on each cheek.

Likewise, never wear a blusher that fights with your lip colour (orange lipstick works better with peach cheeks than pink does, for example); instead of looking naturally beautiful, you will only draw unwanted attention to your artifice.

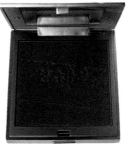

BLUSHER 'RULES'

FAIR-SKINNED women look lovely in pink and tawny tones.

OLIVE-SKINNED/ASIAN TONES look best in brown and copper shades.

BLACK SKINS look great in brighter colours – try plum, fuchsia, deep bronze and warm apricots.

REDHEADS look gorgeous in peach and coral shades, which flatter a typical redhead complexion.

know your face shape

The key to successful application is to know your face well. It is vital to flatter your bone structure (or create the illusion of visible cheekbones) with blusher, but what is the best way to do that? Keep it simple.

THE 'APPLE' APPLICATION

1 With any successful make-up application, you can only work with what you have. In other words, you can make the most of your features, but, without resorting to the surgeon's knife, you cannot completely change them. If you have very full, round cheeks, resist the temptation to 'draw on' cheek bones with excessive shaders and highlighters. The best way to enhance what nature gave you is to stick to the 'apple' application, which is easy to achieve and always looks good.

2 Stand in front of the mirror and smile. Touch the rounded 'pillow' area created when you do this, and consider this your starting point.

3 If using powder blush, dip your brush into the product, then blow off any excess powder. Whip the brush round in even, circular motions, and build up colour slowly to the density required.

4 Stop smiling, then move the brush up and down to create an even 'fade-out'.

5 If using cream blush, apply it to your fingertips, and use similar circular application motions on your cheeks. Make sure that you blend very well.

6 To unite the features, and create the illusion of looking younger, dab blusher across your forehead, nose and chin, to reflect light.

SOFTENING SHARP CHEEKBONES

For those with cheekbones sharper than their eyesight, a slightly different set of rules applies.

1 To make the most of the advantage nature gave you, it may be worth practising a little shading and highlighting. Using the blusher sparingly, applying it well and blending carefully, this effect will add definition to your face. But only use this technique at night, as it will look glaringly obvious natural daylight.

2 When you are using blusher to shade and highlight your cheeks, it is easiest to use powder colour. If possible, use different brushes to apply the product and to blend. Choose colours that are from the same family (for example, a lighter and a darker pink, rather than shades that are startlingly different from each other), as this will create a more natural and more modern look.

3 Remember that dark colours shade and make areas recede – use your deeper tone in the hollows of the cheeks to accentuate their depth. A trick to keep the whole thing looking natural is also to shade the temples, under the chin and down the sides of your nose.

4 If you shade, you must also highlight for balance. So, using the lighter cheek colour, gently sweep over the apples of your cheeks and under the eye socket across your brow bone, and add a little dab to the centre of your chin.

5 This method does require a lot of practice to get it absolutely right. Don't give up after your first attempt, but take care not to leave the house with a stripy face either.

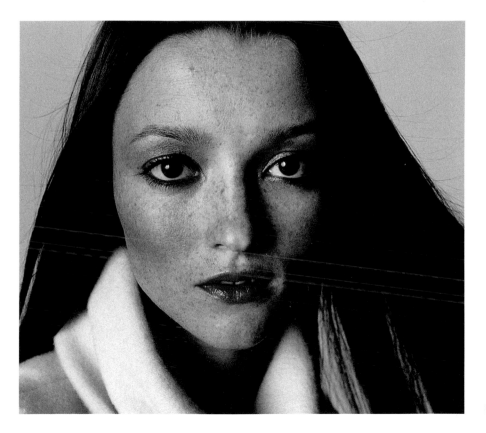

APPLICATION TIPS

1 Always apply powder blush over foundation, or at least powder, and not directly onto bare skin, as this creates a bright, unnatural look and makes it difficult to apply the product smoothly.

2 Do not be afraid to experiment – many a canny beauty sweeps her blusher down her cleavage or along her hairline for a natural, healthy look.

3 A great way to ensure you do not apply too much powder blush to your cheeks is to opt for a brush with white bristles. If your brush looks far too pink, you can be sure your cheeks will, too.

4 Do not panic if you overdo it – tone down colour with translucent powder.

5 Always smile when applying blusher, so that you can locate the cushiony 'apple' of your cheek. Apply blusher here and slanting backwards to your cheekbone.

6 Use your initiative – remember that a touch of lipstick dabbed lightly on the cheeks with the fingertips and properly blended can create a very effective blush.

7 Bear in mind that cream and liquid blushers are kinder to ageing skins. If, like many older women, you suffer from broken veins, a cream blusher, mixed with a little concealer and gently applied in sheer layers, works wonders.

bronzers

Untainted by the long history of traditional blusher (which some still deem old-fashioned), bronzer is a smart way to create a sun-kissed look without exposing your skin to sun damage. Just a whisper, brushed lightly over the cheeks with a voluminous brush, will give you the all-natural, outdoorsy glow of a Ralph Lauren model in a matter of seconds. Also, unlike blusher application, putting on bronzer is virtually foolproof.

Today's bronzers are a more sophisticated breed than the glow-in-the-dark orange products of yesterday. Available in shades to suit everyone from English rose to Asian beauty, bronzers now come in different textures, too. The classic powder form works wonders dusted lightly over the face with a powder brush, while gels, cream and skin tints that wash off with your make-up offer a more moist approach to colour – these tend to reflect more light and hence come closer to the appearance of natural skin. A plethora of wonderful shimmery sticks abound, ensuring you instantly ooze sex when bronzer is stroked over shoulder blades, backs and décolletage.

Bronzer gives you that just-been-on-holiday look, so apply the rest of your make-up accordingly. Lashings of black mascara and a slaver of Vaseline over smooth lips are all you need.

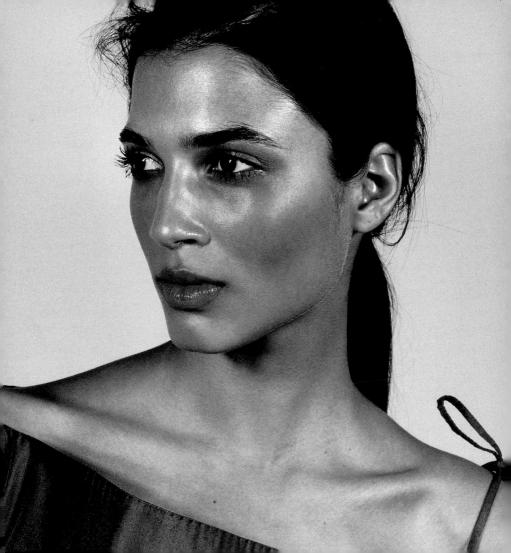

A SAFE TAN IS A FAKE TAN

Whatever the warnings about the dangers of the sun, there is no denying that we all feel better with a suntan – or at least the appearance of one. Rather than lying out like a frying sausage and exposing yourself to the ageing (UVA) and burning (UVB) effects of harmful rays, you are far better off indulging in one of the latest fake tans: these will give you all the benefits of a week-in-the-Caribbean complexion, without exposing you to the associated risks. Thanks to technological developments, today's fake tans are as convincing as the real thing. No more chemical stench, no more streaking and no more orange glow. Today, the tan in a can is available in light, medium and dark tones, as well as in liquid, foam and gel formulations (not to mention tablets that encourage your skin to produce more melanin to deepen its colour). The sexy, sun-kissed look is there for the taking – what's more, you can now enjoy a healthy year-round colour without exposing your skin to harmful rays.

1 Because of the rapidly expanding holes in the ozone layer, sun protection has never been more important than it is today. Even in the cloudiest of winter weather, you should protect your skin with a product with SPF (most decent moisturizers contain one anyway), and never leave home without applying it.

BRONZING TIPS

1 Remember that bronzing powder can double up as eyeshadow.

2 Dust bronzer gently round the hairline to create a natural look.

3 Never choose a bronzer that is darker than your chest colour.

4 Blend, blend, blend into your jaw line to avoid creating a 'seam'.

5 Apply bronzer on top of foundation or powder to be certain of a non-streaky finish.

2 When choosing a fake tan for your face, opt for one that is one shade lighter than your chest to make it look natural (a sun-invoked tan is always lighter on the face than on the body).

3 Make sure the fake tan is intended for facial use. You can use a facial tanner on your body, but not necessarily vice versa.

4 Always do a patch test the night before to make sure you like the colour. The side of the face below the ear and towards the jaw line is the least noticeable place to test.

5 First exfoliate your face thoroughly, and gently, with a facial exfoliating cream or a damp flannel. This will slough off any old skin cells from the surface of the skin and promote a smooth application.

6 If you are worried about the strength of your fake tan, you can always mix it with a moisturizer to lighten its effect.

7 Be especially careful around bony areas such as the nose, as fake tan tends to cling here and you do not want a patchy finish.

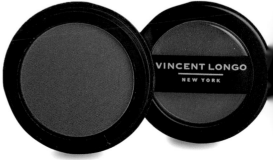

8 Blend well around the jaw line to avoid unnatural demarcation.

9 Use a foundation sponge to apply fake tan if you fear you may not achieve an even coating with your fingertips.

10 Select a fake tan that already has a colour in its cream form, to make sure you can see exactly where you are applying it.

11 If you have oily or acne-prone skin, opt for a product that is oil-free, or a gel that disappears into the skin, leaving just colour, not residue.

SHIMMER

One of the newest trends to infiltrate make-up is shimmer. If you do not fancy coating your cheeks in colour, but want just a subtle wash of sexy sparkle, there are umpteen products that will give you anything from a muted glow to an all-out shine. One trick favoured by make-up artists is to apply natural eyeshadow with a pearlized finish on the cheeks. This acts like a highlighter and gives the skin a subtle sheen. Ultra-sparkly products such as Huile Prodigieuse d'Or by Nuxe look just as good on sun-kissed cheeks as they do rubbed lightly into décolletage and shoulder blades. Alternatively, apply a touch of BeneFit's High Beam to brow bones or cheekbones for a subtle iridescent shimmer.

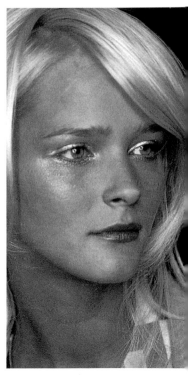

MULTIPURPOSE

Multipurpose make-up has taken the beauty world by storm. Ever since François Nars came up with his marvellous Multiple stick, journalists and fashion aficionados alike have given it all the cult status of a revolutionary discovery. But it is clever marketing, not an entirely new concept, that has so successfully caught the mood of the moment. By the same token, a suitable shade of lipstick will work just as well smudged into your cheeks and eyelids as products labelled for those specific applications. Use your initiative, and apply your favourite make-up products wherever they look good.

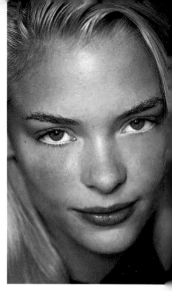

DEWY CHEEKS

No wonder 'light-reflecting' make-up causes such excitement. The dewy complexion of youth, once lost, is incredibly hard to recapture, and any cosmetic enhancement is a welcome addition to our make-up bags. Look for foundations and blushers that contain 'light-reflecting particles' – these refract the light and bounce it off the face, giving an instant boost to a dull complexion. You do not need to invest in a new foundation to create a dewy look – any pearlized blusher or bronzer will give a similar effect and can be kinder to mature skins. Remember that powder, cream and gel formulations can all create the same effect – the secret is to go pearlized and avoid anything too matt (and therefore ageing). If you are slightly tanned, Vaseline rubbed lightly over the cheeks and mouth gives a deliciously sensual twist to a dewy complexion.

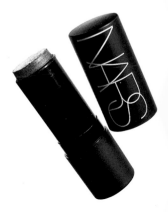

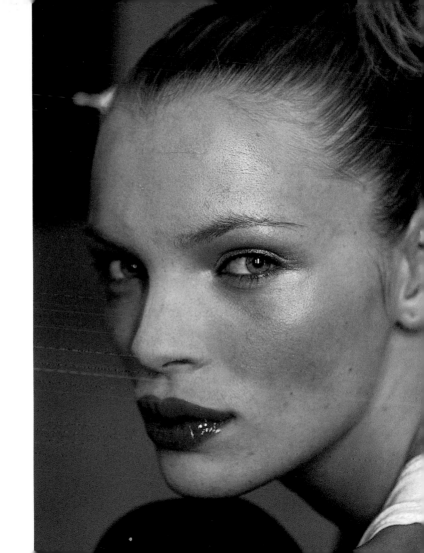

THE AUDREY
(OR HOW TO CREATE GAMINE CHIC)

1 Apply liquid concealer in tiny dots around any unsightly under-eye circles. Concealer should always be at least a couple of shades lighter than the skin.

2 Next, take a soft brown eye pencil, sharp but with the end smoothed off slightly, to define the eyebrow. You can extend the line above the eyebrow, but never below it if you wish to maintain a natural look. Make sure that the part of the brow nearest the nose is the thickest, thinning out slightly towards the top of the curve, then tapering out towards the outer corner of the eye. But take care not to exaggerate this or you will end up with a 'tadpole' look.

3 Now take an eyeshadow brush, and apply a wash of neutral powder eyeshadow to both the eyelids. Take this no further than the crease of your eye (which appears when your eyes are open). Next, using a gentle, fingertip application, apply a neutral cream eyeshadow from the crease line right up to the eyebrow, being sure to blend especially well where it meets the powder eyeshadow.

4 Take a clear mascara and, using the wand, sweep the eyebrow hairs gently upwards. This gives the eyebrows a natural, just-groomed look.

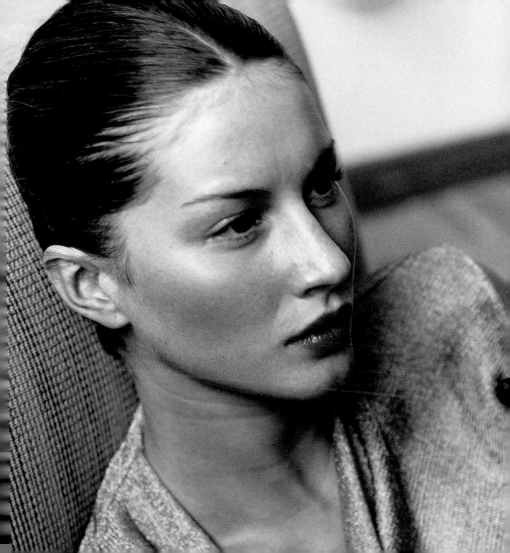

5 Curl the eyelashes using a good eyelash curler. Make sure that you keep the pressure even along the entire length of the lashes so that you don't create a sharp bend. Apply dark mascara to top and bottom lashes.

6 Use an eyelash comb to separate the top lashes before the mascara has dried, and apply another coat if you need to.

7 Next, take your blusher brush, and, using gentle circular motions, apply a touch of pale pink blusher to the apples of the cheeks only. Start with just a little – you can always add another layer of blush to create more depth later.

8 Define your mouth by lining it with a flesh-toned lip pencil, which should be quite sharp, but not too pointed. Fill in the whole area using the same pencil (so that you are not left with an unnatural outline a couple of hours down the road), and finish with a coat of transparent gloss or Vaseline on top of the lip liner colour.

THE MARILYN
(OR HOW TO ENSURE GENTLEMEN PREFER BLONDES)

1 This look is based on making the most of your eyes and your lips. Take a concealer a couple of shades paler than the one you normally use, and dot it around the under-eye area.

2 Rim your eyes with white or beige pencil, which will make the whites of your eyes appear whiter. Make sure the pencil is soft-edged before your start and apply to top and bottom lids by gently lifting them with your fingers.

3 Using a soft, beige eyeshadow, blend carefully right up to the brow bone. Next, highlight from the crease of the eye up to the brow bone with a pearlized white shadow.

4 Using a smoky brown eye pencil, sweep one continuous line across top and bottom lashes, as close to the edge as possible, so that there is no visible line of skin between the eye pencil and the lashes. Do not buff this line with the rubber-tipped hoof.

5 Using a professional eyelash curler, curl back your eyelashes. (Remember to 'step' the curler out along the full length of your lashes to avoid an unnatural bend.) Carefully apply black mascara, thickening it slightly towards the outer edges.

6 Stick to pale pink, rather than a peach, blusher for a starker look. This can also be used along the hair line and under your chin to create the illusion of a rosy reflection. Using a blunt-edged brown eyeliner, draw a beauty spot at the side of one cheek, roughly midway between your nose and lips.

7 Line your lips with a red lip pencil. (Blue reds work better with pink blusher than yellow reds here.) Fill in with a creamy, true red lipstick (YSL has an unbeatable range), blot your lips and reapply. For a really seductive finish, coat the mouth generously with Clarins' clear lip gloss.

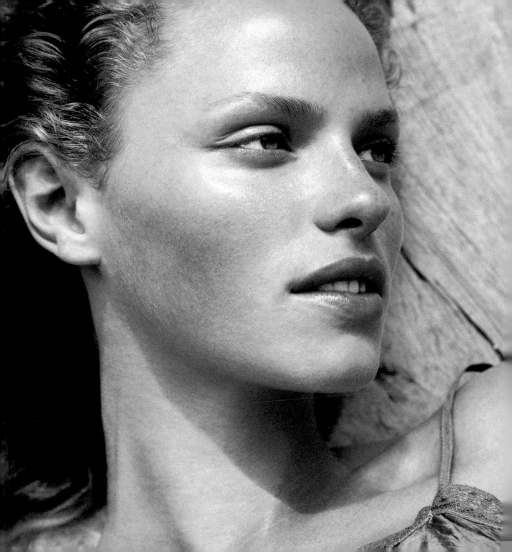

NATURALLY BEAUTIFUL
(OR HOW TO COMBAT REALITY)

1 Choose a stick foundation in a shade that blends imperceptibly with your natural skin tone, and apply it to the nose, eyelids, forehead and around your mouth. Do not feel that you have to cover any other areas of the face with foundation – the aim here is to look as natural as possible.

2 Next, apply a tiny amount of liquid highlighter about one shade lighter than the foundation you have chosen down the nose and around your mouth. Blend it in very well, particularly in the nose area, otherwise the foundation can tend to sit rather obviously around the larger pores on this part of your face.

3 Choose a voluminous face brush, and dip it luxuriantly into a pot of translucent loose powder. Apply the powder all over the face, being especially generous in the under-eye area (this will help to catch any stray pigments that may fall from the eyelids later in step 5).

4 Fill in any patchy bits of eyebrow with an eyebrow pencil one shade lighter than your brows, making sure that you use broken movements to keep a natural line.

5 Take a pale beige cream eyeshadow, with just a hint of shimmer, and, using your fingertips, blend it from the lash line right up to meet the brow bone. Now carefully brush away any excess powder from underneath your eyes.

6 Avoid eyeliner, as this makes people realize that you are wearing make-up – defeating the purpose of looking 'naturally beautiful'. Instead, curl your lashes as always, and apply a single coat of dark brown (not black) mascara.

7 Use a flesh-coloured lip liner (MAC's Spice is the supermodels' favourite) to trace the natural outline of your lips. Fill in your mouth using the same colour, then, using a pale, peachy-pink shade, brush a creamy lipstick over the entire mouth area. Avoid matt shades, as these look less natural. Blot and reapply.

8 Lastly, using a blusher brush (do not use a powder brush), apply a light dusting of pale pink or apricot blusher to the apples of your cheeks only (see the tips on pages 242–3 for how best to achieve this).

SHIMMER
(OR HOW TO APPLY FROSTED PRODUCTS WITHOUT LOOKING LIKE A 1970s THROWBACK)

1 Apply under-eye concealer as in the previous looks.

2 Apply your foundation in the usual way, blending well with either the fingertips or a make-up sponge.

3 Next, using as voluminous a brush as possible, add a whisper of translucent powder over your foundation to set it.

4 Using your fingertips, apply a neutral, matt cream eye-

shadow as a base colour. This should be washed right from the lash line up to the brow bone. Make sure you blend very well, as this shadow will act as a base coat for your glitter products.

5 Now outline your eyes with a dark eye pencil, or a dark shadow, applied in a thin line with a tiny brush.

6 Choose a powder eyeshadow with a high-frost finish, in any colour (metallic colours look the least retro). Smudge the shadow onto the brow bone, just below the eyebrow, tapering out towards the eyelid crease. This opens up the eye.

7 Alternatively, you can use real glitter for the disco-diva look, but this requires absolute precision of application, as you cannot blend real glitter without spreading it everywhere. If you do choose this option, be prepared to find glitter around your house for weeks afterwards.

8 Next, curl your eyelashes carefully, and apply mascara to top and bottom lashes. Comb the top lashes out before you apply a second coat.

9 Take a lip liner several shades darker than your chosen lip colour. Outline your lips carefully, blending the colour inwards onto the lips themselves.

10 Fill in the lips with a frosted lipstick. Coat with a clear lip gloss or a lick of Vaseline, and, for added shine, sprinkle glitter in the centre of the cupid's bow and the bottom lip.

TOO HOT TO HANDLE
(OR HOW TO LOOK LIKE A SEX KITTEN)

1 Apply under-eye concealer, foundation and powder as in the previous looks.

2 Using a voluminous brush, dust a generous helping of loose translucent powder on the bridge of your nose, under the eyes and on your chin.

3 Next, use an eyebrow pencil one shade lighter than your natural lashes (never go darker) to fill in any patchy sections. Use a series of light, broken brushstrokes to keep the line looking natural. Brush the eyebrow hairs upwards with an eyebrow brush. Trim any stray hairs very carefully using a pair of sharp nail scissors.

4 Blend a beige cream eyeshadow into the eyelid, up to where the crease forms when your eyes are open.

5 With a firm, medium-sized eyeshadow brush, apply a coat of white frosted-powder shadow, starting at your lash line and going right up to the eyebrow. Sweep it generously towards the outer corners of your eyes. Do not worry if the shimmer ends up straying beyond the corners – this will only add to your allure.

6 With a steady hand, apply black kohl pencil to the upper eyelids, keeping the line close to the lashes. Have the pencil as sharp as possible and make one continuous action. (This

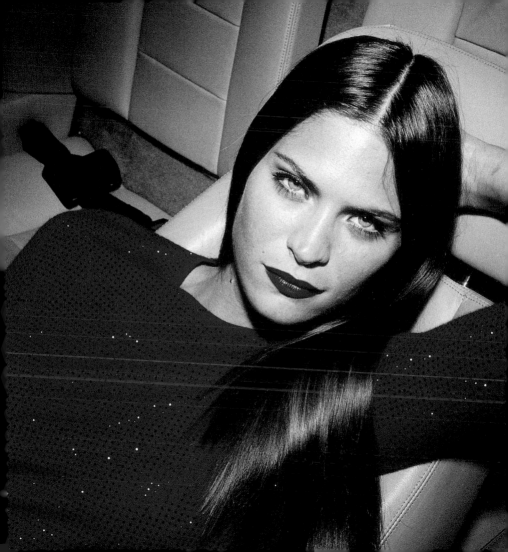

takes a lot of practice, so make sure you have mastered it before a big night out.) Slope the line down and then let it flick up slightly at the corners for a 'come to bed' look.

7 Curl the lashes with an eyelash curler, then apply black mascara to the top and bottom lashes. After brushing the top lashes carefully, apply a second coat.

8 When the mascara has dried, use a thin eyeshadow brush to draw a line of shadow under the eyes, sloping down to the outer corners to match the upper lids.

9 Using a good blusher brush, sweep a pinkish blusher upwards on your cheeks, following the line of the cheekbones rather than concentrating on the 'apple'.

10 Line the lips with a red pencil, going slightly outside the natural lip line (make sure your mouth is relaxed). Using the same liner, lightly colour the lips to make sure you are not left with an unnatural outline when your lipstick wears off.

11 Fill in the lips with pure red lipstick. Blot, reapply and then add lip gloss or Vaseline to complete the siren look.

THE BRIGHT SPARK
(OR HOW TO WEAR COLOUR AND LOOK STUNNING)

1 Apply under-eye concealer, foundation and powder in the previous looks. Then line the top and bottom eyelids with blue eyeliner – the darker your eyes, the deeper the blue.

2 Using an eyeshadow brush, apply a blue eyeshadow that is about two shades lighter than the liner to the top eyelids. Start from the lash line and blend out until it reaches just above the crease. Also add a little colour underneath the eye. Blend well so that the colour fades naturally.

3 Next, apply a beige liquid eyeshadow to the centre of the lids and blend in well so that the colour appears graduated.

4 Curl your eyelashes and apply mascara, brushing the top lashes (before they dry) before the second application.

5 Apply coloured gloss or lip stain to your lips. Do not outline your lips or you will end up looking like a caricature. If you have used blue eye colour, stick to a blue-based lip colour (anything from pale pink to red would look effective).

6 Remember that you can always vary the blue eye colour with a different hue entirely. Follow the same principle for green, say, by keeping the shadow lighter than the liner and sticking to an orange-based lipstick (in any shade from coral to carrot), rather than a blue-based one.

7 For a more outdoorsy finish, blend cream blusher into the cheekbones. (Use pink blush with blue shadow, and apricot blush with green shadow.)

SMOKY AND SMOULDERING

1 Apply under-eye concealer, foundation and powder as in previous looks. Then, using a white eye pencil, line the inner rim of the eyes, top and bottom.

2 Apply chocolate-brown eyeshadow along the crease line only, starting at the outer corner of the eye and working inwards towards the nose.

3 Using eyeshadow a shade lighter, smudge a line beneath your lower lashes.

4 Next, use a fine brush to apply a line of black eyeshadow to the upper lash line. Smudge it into the chocolate shadow in the crease of the eye.

5 Curl your lashes, then apply lashings of black mascara (which should be combed before it dries) and, when it has dried, add a second coat.

6 Using a claret lip pencil, trace slightly outside the natural lip line. Fill in with the same pencil, and then fill with a deep red lipstick. Blot, reapply and cover with a natural lip gloss.

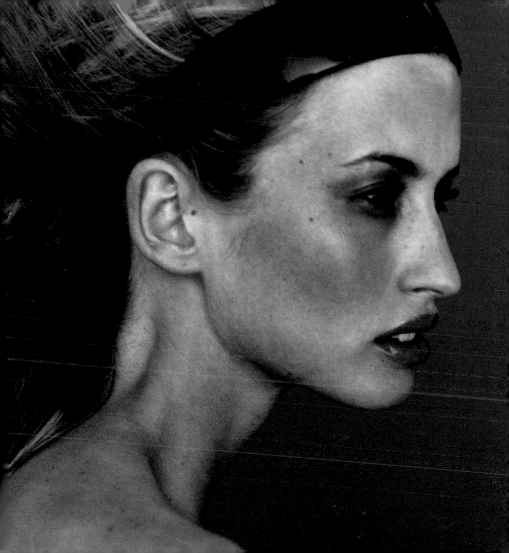

DEWY-FACED

1 Apply concealer one shade lighter than your foundation under the eyes, as before.

2 Next, using a 'light-reflective' (not a matt) foundation, apply base over the entire face, blending well with the fingertips. Mix it first with a pearlized primer (such as Lancôme's Maquisuperbe) and, starting at the centre of the face, blend carefully outwards.

3 Taking an apricot cream blusher with a pearlized finish, smile and apply blusher to the apples of the cheeks only.

4 Use a high-sheen cream eyeshadow in a brown tone over the eyelid, sweeping colour just above the crease line. Next, blend in an ivory pearlized eyeshadow from the crease line to the brow bone.

5 Brush your eyebrows upwards with an eyebrow comb, and fill in any patches with an eyebrow pencil one shade lighter than your natural eyebrow colour. Make broken, feathery movements to do this.

6 Curl your lashes carefully, taking pains not to create a sharp bend, and apply dark brown mascara to the top lashes only.

7 Line the lips with a pinky-peach liner, and fill in with the same colour.

8 Coat the lips with a clear lip gloss.

9 For really exaggerated shine, use an eye gloss (Calvin Klein makes a great one) or Vaseline to cover the eyelids. Although this is not as long-lasting as a high-shimmer powder, it looks very effective in the short term.

10 Brush a glittery bronzer over the shoulder blades and décolletage to complete the look.

CELEBRITY SECRETS (ELIZABETH HURLEY'S 5-MINUTE MAKE-UP)

1 I start with a scrupulously clean and well-moisturized face. I always begin with my eyes first and start by concealing any dark shadows.

2 Then I use a soft brown eye pencil and draw smudgy lines close to the lashes, top and bottom. I blend these further with a brush, which I have dipped in a gleamy brown powder shadow. This stops the eye pencil from running during the day; powder alone will not last.

3 I curl my lashes and apply black mascara. After pencilling in my eyebrows, I set them with brow gel so that they do not rebel during the day.

4 Next, I use a light stick foundation, which I blend with my fingers, and then a stick blush in pink, which I also blend very well. I use a very small amount of loose powder just to set the foundation, as I loathe seeing powder on the skin.

5 For lips, I first use a pencil and then one of Estée Lauder's lipsticks, which make your lips look huge.

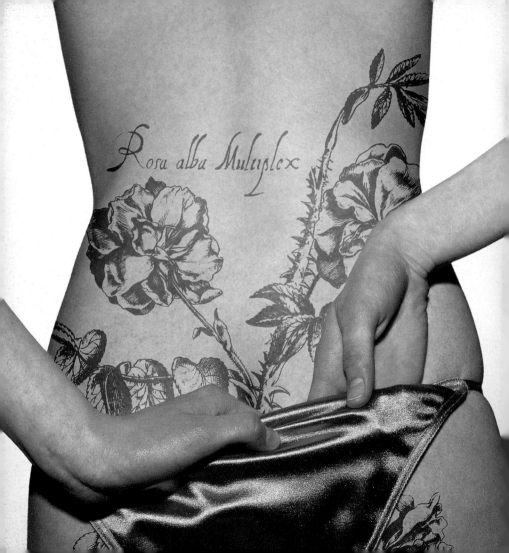

7 body & hair

'Love your body. A natural part of loving your body is looking after it.'
Theresa Hale, Hale Clinic

'Clean, shiny hair is a joy to have and head-turning to watch.'
Charles Worthington, celebrity hairdresser

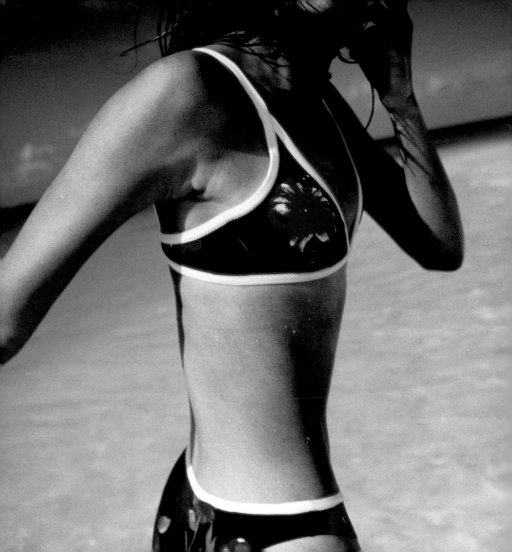

Learn to love your body and you will feel a whole lot better about yourself. Believe it or not, far more women are unhappy with their body shape than with their faces – despite the fact that the body is covered up for most of the time. Achieving 'media-perceived' perfection (a minute dress size) is ultimately unattainable for most of us, so rather than wasting time trying to achieve unrealistic goals, channel your positive energy into accepting your size and shape, and aim to be the best possible you, rather than a different you altogether. After all, it is more often the quality of our skin, not the quantity (or lack of it) that counts. Think back to Sophie Dahl, with her smooth alabaster curves wrapped tantalizingly around the advertising slogans for Parfums YSL. What strikes you is the milky perfection of her skin, its flawless luminosity and unblemished texture.

While the benefits of studio lighting and air brushing are not available to all of us, there is still a lot we can do to keep our bodies in shape, and our skin in peak condition. Small lifestyle improvements (doing more exercise to improve muscle and skin tone, and drinking more water to flush toxins from the system, for example) go a long way in the quest for self-improvement. While you may not end up gracing the next fragrance campaign in your birthday suit, you will certainly look, and feel, a lot better.

GOOD SKIN DIET

1 Drink an average of eight glasses of water a day.

2 Eat natural vegetable oils (especially olive oil) and fish oils, which are wonderful for the skin and beneficial to the metabolism.

3 Eat plenty of fruit and vegetables. These contain natural sugars and will give you long-lasting energy.

4 Drink plenty of freshly squeezed, diluted fruit juice for a turbo boost of vitamins and to improve the appearance of your skin.

skincare

Most of us spend hours worrying about our silhouettes, yet we tend to neglect the texture of our skin, which also plays a vital part in the way we look. Dedicate just a few extra minutes to looking after your body at bath time, and you will be amazed at the results.

1 During the winter months your body spends most of its time swaddled in layers of clothing. You flit from freezing temperatures outside to centrally heated atmospheres inside without thinking of the havoc this wreaks on your system. Cell renewal slows down, and old, flaky skin cells accumulate, leading to a grey, lacklustre appearance. Exfoliate at least once a week, using either a long-handled loofah (which will help you reach those difficult parts, such as your back) or an exfoliating body scrub (Clinique's is my clear favourite).

2 Bony areas, such as knees and elbows, need extra attention. Use a deeply moisturizing agent (such as petroleum jelly) to keep knees and elbows soft and young-looking.

3 Avoid taking very hot baths and showers – these can lead to broken capillaries. Cool baths and showers help boost the circulation and 'wake up' the skin, leaving you fresh and rejuvenated.

4 Stand up and be counted. Bad posture means your body is out of alignment, and can never look its best. Hold your shoulders and neck back, keep your chin and eyes up and till your pelvis slightly towards the front. This simple corrective can add inches to your height, and make all the difference to your appearance.

5 Remember to slather any exposed areas of your body with sun protection at all times, even in midwinter. Sun exposure is the single most important factor in premature skin ageing.

6 Moisturize every time you have a bath. Dry skin wrinkles on your body just as it does on your face. Change the strength of your moisturizer according to the seasons – if you are on the beach, in the sand and in the sea, you will need more protection.

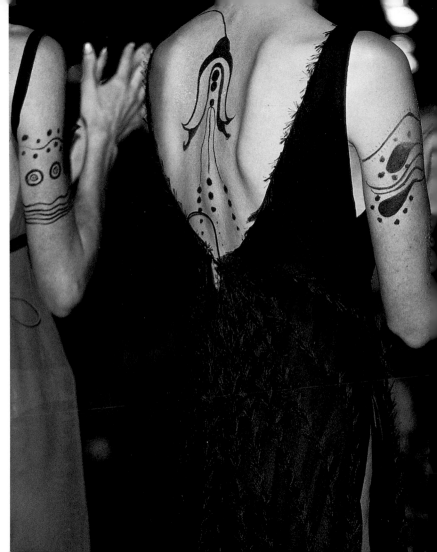

body make-up

Once the sole domain of tribal warriors, Hell's Angels, and famous show-offs (think Demi Moore's painted birthday suit in *Vanity Fair* magazine), body art is now so mainstream you almost make more of a statement without it. Thanks to designers like Alexander McQueen and Julien Macdonald (who sent models down recent runways with spiky nails, bejewelled bodies and rainbow coloured hair), and modern beauty icons such as Angelina Jolie with her tattooed torso, the fashion for donning a temporary bindi or tattoo to totally turning yourself into a piece of walking art, has broken down the boundaries of class and culture.

While head-to-toe body painting is beauty's answer to wearing a couture dress (and no girl worth her Mehndi paste would consider attempting it without the talents of a professional make-up artist to hand), there are other ways to adorn your body which do not require the same investment of time or money. On the shelves of every department store (not to mention your local pharmacy) are a glittering array of sparkling gels, pearlescent creams and shimmering lotions which, spread between your shoulder blades or across your décolletage, serve as seductive aids to cosmetic enhancement, drawing attention to every inch of flesh you dare to bare.

Mehndi kits and self-adhesive bindis add an ethnic edge to body decoration, (even Madonna is a fan of these – check out the henna designs she sported in her 'Ray of Light' video), while temporary tattoos in shapes as diverse as girlie hearts to intricate flower designs are an alternative way to liven up your wrists, your ankles, or the nape of your neck. For all those bright sparks out there, body jewels offer a great way make sure you really shine out. The navel is an obvious place to twinkle, but coloured gemstones also look great twisted around the upper arm, snuggled around the ankle, or even glued delicately to the side of your nose.

Body art is a great way to experiment with colour for those who prefer to keep their make-up neutral. A technicolour tattoo will liven up your jeans and white T-shirt, while a flash of ruby, a glimmer of emerald, or a touch of tourmaline sparkling against a simple black dress will effectively turn your look from classic cocktail to erotic siren.

A NEW CANVAS

Changing demographics and the growing influence of ethnic fashion have helped to spread make-up beyond the face. The body has become the new canvas for decoration – from jewels to temporary and permanent tattoos to intricate henna designs. Whether you want something that will make you stand out for a special occasion, or decide to go for a more lasting signature, is up to you. Here are some of the many types of body art that are now available:

SPARKLE

Sparkle and glitter add a modern twist to the classic body moisturizer. Try Huile Prodigieuse d'Or by Nuxe, with its shimmering particles, on décolletage and shoulder blades; or if you really feel like going for gold, Guerlain makes a body cream containing real gold glitter. Glitter products are also available in mousse and gel forms; these tend to soak in completely, leaving just a sparkle on the skin. Real glitter can also be used (stick it in place with eyelash glue) to create pretty patterns on the face or body, and add instant glamour to your look.

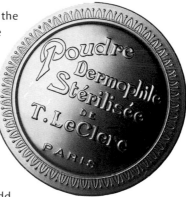

PIERCING

Once, piercing your nose was seen as a sign of rebellion – my, how times have changed. Without wishing to list the somewhat varied and imaginative locations that today's 'earrings' find themselves in, I will simply point out the modern rule of thumb: if you fancy an unconventional piercing, and have a high pain threshold, do it – but always go to a reputable piercer.

TATTOOS

A seriously downmarket signifier in the past, in recent years the tattoo has broken the barriers of class and culture, and taken a firm seat at the forefront of fashion. Tattoos now range from something as subtle as a gentle line to enhance the lashes or the lip shape, to huge, intricate works of art in a multitude of different designs and colours, and celebrity endorsement has ensured they are here to stay.

These days the process can involve anything from following a stencil pattern to inspired freehand work. If you do decide to go freehand, make sure you like the work of the artist before you bare your flesh. Word of mouth is the best way to discover a reliable salon (tattooing no longer necessitates entering a grimy booth on the sea front), but, needless to say, always check the hygiene, antiseptic and anaesthetic standards first.

TEMPORARY TATTOOS

For those who do not want anything permanent, temporary tattoos mean you can enjoy the effect without the pain or the longevity of the real thing.

1 Temporary tattoo inks usually come in a kit containing several colours and a brush (temporary tattoo pens are also available for easy application).

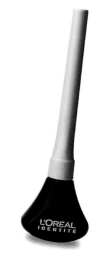

2 As it is thinner than standard body paint, you need to apply tattoo ink in layers to build up intensity.

3 Practise using tattoo stamps, which is not as easy at it sounds: too much ink and the pattern will smudge, too little and it will be barely noticeable.

4 For those more interested in the ends than the means, tattoo transfers provide the ideal answer. Bands look great around the wrist or ankle, and the outlines can always be painted in with body paint if you are feeling arty. Tattoo transfers can be removed easily with baby oil.

A GIRL'S BEST FRIEND

No abdomen toned to the standards of Jessica Alba is complete without a sparkling navel. Cropped tops, low-slung skirts and hipster trousers are ideal for the look, which calls for no more than a fake jewel and a blob of glue. Celebrities including Madonna, Demi Moore and Helena Christensen made the 'bindi', or body jewel, de rigueur for physical enhancement. Worn traditionally by Indian women to show that they are married, bindis range from the simplest solo spot to astonishingly complex designs.

Authentic self-adhesive bindis are available from Indian shops and supermarkets, but the current trend means that fashionable alternatives are easily found in

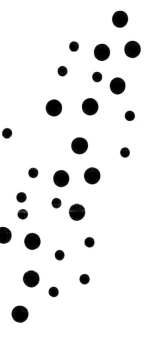

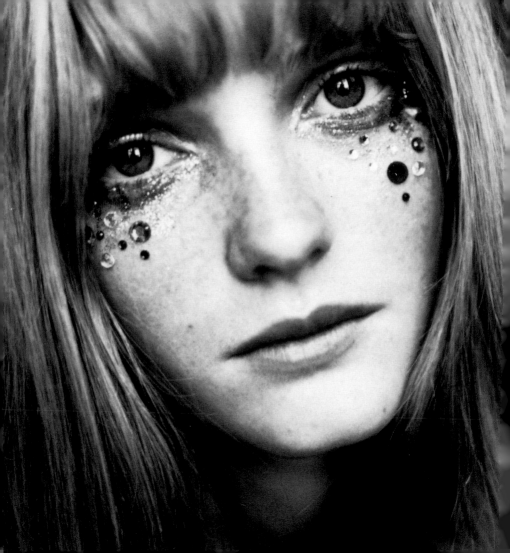

many department stores. Wear them between the eyes, above the arch of the eyebrow, around your wrists, ankles or shoulders – all you need are the bindis, or jewels, and some eyelash glue.

BODY JEWELS

1 Choose a bindi or diamanté body jewel to match the colour of your clothing.

2 Glittery make-up looks terrific with diamanté or crystal bindis.

3 When fixing a bindi between the eyebrows make sure it is centred and slightly higher than the brow line. If it is pointed, keep the point facing upwards towards the hairline.

4 Try using a bindi as a nose stud.

5 Add a sparkle to your eyes by sticking tiny diamantés all along your lash line with eyelash glue.

6 If using traditional kumkum powder with a stencil, remember to cover the skin in eyelash glue first, and then paint the kumkum over it. This will hold it in place.

7 Always apply a bindi after you have finished your make-up.

8 Bindis can be kept and reused. Self-adhesive ones can always be stuck on with false eyelash glue if their sticky backing wears off.

STENCILS

Artistically minded babes will find that traditional body painting is a great way to express individual style. You can choose from either metal or cardboard stencils (available from specialist Indian shops, as before) and from a variety of paint textures. Body paints are normally used to fill in stencils, but liquid eyeliner or lipstick applied with a fine-tipped brush will do much the same job. If you really want to glow for it, ultraviolet paints show up brilliantly in club lighting. Designs such as butterflies, stars, hearts and flowers are always pretty; these can be used alone, or repeated as a decorative motif around the wrist, for example.

BODY PAINT

Body paint is a good temporary alternative to a tattoo. Whether you decide to cover a large surface area with an intricate image, or just want to draw attention to a flash of exposed shoulder or décolletage, all you need are some paints, a brush and a lot of practice. Remember that body paints, like any form of make-up, can cause allergic reactions on some skins, so always do a small patch test before you paint large areas.

1 Water-based body paints are readily available in a rainbow of bright colours. Avoid using children's face paints if you want to save your clothes, as they tend to be rather greasy and slide around.

2 Dust the area to be painted with translucent powder before you start. This will keep the finished design in place, and stop the paint moving on your skin while you are painting.

3 If you are painting an image with several colours, make sure that each colour has dried properly before you start to apply the next.

4 If you want to blend the colours, apply them in sequence while they are still wet and mix thoroughly.

5 If you dare to paint freehand, draw on the design first with a white eyeliner, then trace over it with colour.

6 Body paints can be removed either with soap and water, or with your normal facial cleanser.

7 Remember that some body paints double up as nail paints – which will save you money as well as cabinet space. Nail varnishes, however, do not double up as body paints.

8 Body paints also come in crayon form, making it easier to complete detailed line work, and create sharper edges.

9 Glitter paints can be used to great effect either on their own, or to highlight a matt design.

10 If you are using stencils for your designs, keep them in place on your skin with masking tape.

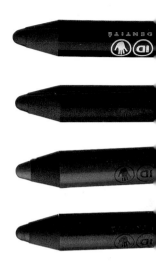

MEHNDI

Mehndi, or henna painting, has been used for centuries to adorn the hands and feet of Indian brides. Currently fashionable in the West, Mehndi transfers and pens have made it more accessible, but unlike the authentic henna painting, which fades after three weeks, the ink from these will wash off.

Follow these steps provided by Madonna's mehndi artist, Sumita Batra:

1 To make a staining agent, place a tea bag with 2 tsp instant coffee in a cup. Half fill with water and microwave on high for 20 seconds. Set aside for 20 minutes.

2 Place 1 heaped tbsp fine henna powder in a bowl, then gradually mix in the staining agent to make a smooth paste. Cover and set aside for 24 hours. The paste will keep for about two weeks.

3 Roll a square of plastic into a cone, sealing it with clear tape. The point of the cone should be the size of a pencil point. Tape up the tip and spoon the paste into the cone. Roll down the top of the cone tightly and tape so the cone is filled firmly. Untape the point and practise squeezing henna out in an even line.

4 Draw the design with the prepared henna paste. Leave to dry for 20 minutes.

5 To set design, mix 3 tbsp lemon juice and 1 tbsp sugar. Dab the solution all over the design. Allow to dry. Do not touch. The paste will crumble off over the next few hours, leaving a deep residue of colour.

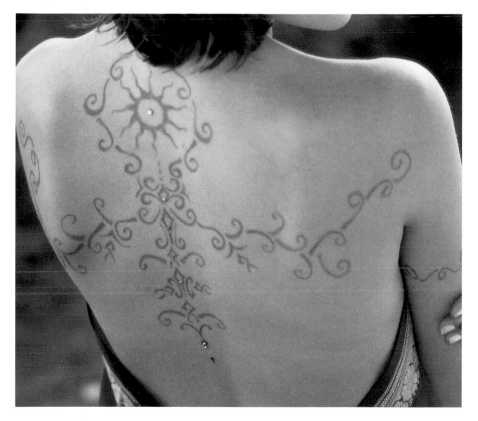

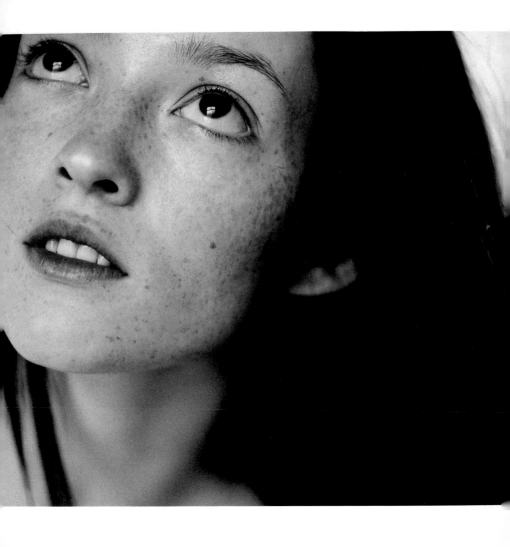

hair make-up

Hair says as much about our personal style and psyche as our choice of make-up or the clothes we wear. It is also a direct barometer of how good we feel about ourselves: if our hair looks great, we approach the day with attitude (quite literally with our head held up); on a bad hair day we feel utter misery and lack of confidence. The cult status of the 'celebrity hairdresser' speaks volumes about the importance of hair to today's women – and explains why Orlando Pita, John Frieda, Nicky Clarke et al. have become household names all over the world.

While having great hair once meant having hair that was shiny, manageable and well cut, today's hair is more about individual statement and expression. Your hair should set you apart from the group, not bind you to it (think 1960s bob worn as an identity badge). Today's star hairdressers are distinguished not so much by a trademark cut as by shaping and enhancing the unique potential of each individual client. 'You have to have a hairstyle that first and foremost suits you,' says John Frieda. 'It has to fit into your timeframe and say who you are.'

Who you are can change on a daily basis, of course. Thanks to the influence of catwalk trends on today's hairstyles, it is now possible to go from gamine crop to Rapunzel-like tresses overnight (à la Victoria Beckham and Gwyneth Paltrow), from blonde to red and back again in a couple of washes, and from dressed down to tressed up in a matter of minutes. The only things you need to transform your look are the right tools, the willingness to embrace change, and a little knowledge of what to do and when to do it.

COLOUR

Change your hair colour, and you change the way the world perceives you, not just on a physical level but on a psychological one, too. Just think about it – redheads are traditionally associated with a fiery temper, blondes with bimbo tendencies and brunettes with classic sophistication. Thanks to the technicolour world of temporary hair colour, going from ebony to orange no longer requires a long-term commitment – hair mascaras, gels and sprays can transform your look in milliseconds, and last you all the way from the party to your next hair wash.

COLOURED SPRAYS

These are much easier to use than mascara if you want to cover large areas of hair. For an all-over 'mist' effect, hold the can about 25–30 cm (10–12 in) away from your hair as you spray (stand over a basin, just in case); for blocks of more intense colour, hold the spray about 10 cm (4 in) away from your hair. Metallic spray colours are particularly effective.

COLOURED MOUSSES

Splendid if you want to change your colour just for an evening, coloured mousses also add volume to your hair. 'Always seek professional advice first,' says Charles Worthington, 'as these mousses can leave a colour cast on your hair.'

COLOURED WAXES

Best used in small sections, coloured waxes can add drama to hair for an evening, but watch out if your hair is already bleached, as the colour can enter the hair shaft and stain it.

COLOURED HAIRPIECES

A great way to enjoy the drama of strong colour, without any of the commitment, coloured hair pieces are easily woven into your natural hair, and easily removed without causing any damage.

SEMI-PERMANENT RINSES

These vegetable-based dyes have revolutionized colouring, because they do not contain hydrogen peroxide and are therefore less damaging to the hair. However, they cannot be used to lighten hair, only to add depth to your existing colour. They condition the hair by sealing the cuticle, and thus making a smooth surface for light to bounce off, creating shine. They wash out totally after about ten shampoos. Use a dark towel after washing your hair, as the colour tends to mark when your hair is wet.

COLOUR WASHES

These are exactly what they say – colours that wash in then out in the next shampoo. They are fine if you want to enhance your hair colour for an evening, and do not need lasting commitment.

MASCARA TIPS

Charles Worthington says: 'Always test the colour at the beauty counter first, as a shade that looks pretty in a tube can look pretty dull or unnoticeable in your hair.'

1 Hair mascara looks great if it picks up a colour in your clothing. For a subtle look, apply it at the hairline for a 'highlight' effect.

2 For a more fashion-forward approach, apply the mascara in chunky sections. This technique works especially well on asymmetrical hair styles, and will make you appear bold and outgoing.

3 If you are wearing a tight top, remember to put it on before you apply your hair mascara. This will reduce the risk of staining clothing, even though hair mascara dries quite quickly.

4 Remember to choose a hair mascara to match your make-up – if you are wearing coral lipstick, for example, choose an orange-, not pink-toned, hair mascara.

5 The natural colour of your hair need not be a factor in your choice of hair mascara – think rather the bolder the better. The greater the contrast with your natural hair colour, the more striking the effect will be.

6 Look chic, not streak – always stick to one colour at a time.

HAIR ACCESSORIES

These days every head-turning fashionista knows the power of an eye-catching hair accessory. Thanks to the Johnnie Loves Rosie cult, everything from oversized flowers to feathers to sparkling butterfly clips to iridescent hair jewels will add instant glamour to your overall look. Whether you are wearing a bikini or an evening dress, you will not feel dressed without one.

1 For long hair: turn your hair upside down, roughly dry it and backcomb the underneath for volume. Pull your hair into a tight top knot. Then add a huge flower, either behind the ear secured with a grip, or into the band holding the ponytail. Real flowers look best, but there are bouquets of fake ones to choose from.

2 For short hair: using styling gel (wet-look works well), twist your hair into small peaks all over your head. Use a glittery hair slide right at the front in the centre of your forehead for instant effect.

3 For straight hair: part your hair neatly to one side, then attach jewelled kirby grips at 5-cm (2-in) intervals down the length of your hair, on the opposite side to your parting.

4 For curly hair: scatter sparkling butterfly clips through your hair.

5 For any hair: try some of the marvellous glitter sprays and gels that greet you at every pharmacy and department store. They look wonderful applied around the hairline and down the sides of your hair, and complement the trend for sparkling make-up.

6 Stylist Luke Hersheson says: 'Today it does not matter what shape your face is – you can wear whatever style you like, as long as you wear it with confidence.' And even if nature gave you poker-straight locks, you can always crimp it then strew it with dazzling jewels for an enchanted evening.

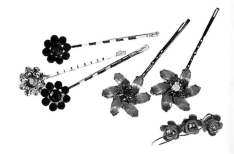

HAIR DRESSING

1 Anywhere clothes can go, hair can often go too, and this applies to the trend for tie-dyeing. Best on mid-length hair, this involves putting vibrant colours on the ends of the hair only, making a drastic contrast with your natural colour. For dark hair, red works brilliantly. Blondes should avoid green, but look striking with gold, silver or dark brown tie-dye.

2 Feel like a redhead trapped in a blonde's hairdo? Show your true colours to most dramatic effect by having the underneath of your hair dyed pillar-box red. This will not show when your hair is au naturel in the office, but tie it up in a high ponytail or chignon at night, and let your fiery character come shining through.

3 Vibrant colours look fantastic in solid blocks. But do not try this at home – visit a salon.

4 Add instant glamour to your hairstyle by spraying glitter along your parting line.

5 Use two colours for a more textured finish. You can either colour the top layers with a deep colour and the underneath layers with a softer shade, or vice versa. Leave this one to the professionals to guarantee a gorgeous result.

6 For the more artistic (or those with very steady hands), a carefully applied stencil is sure to turn heads. Remember that simple, bold shapes work best on hair. Either grip the stencil in place, use gaffer tape (if you do not mind losing a few hairs in the process) or ask a friend to hold it for you. Using a brush and some washable body paint, fill in the design carefully. (Hold the stencil very still to avoid smudging.) While the paint is still wet, sprinkle glitter over the design for added sparkle. Alternatively, forget the body paint and just fill in the stencil with a glitter spray. Keep the spray close to the hair to make sure it does not end up outside the stencil design.

HAIR EXTENSIONS

Once, having long hair required years of patient growing. Today, if a girl wants long hair she can have it now. Creative talent in the haircare industry means that extensions so natural that even you will not be able to tell them apart from your own locks are readily available at most salons. If you tire of your gamine crop, all you need are a couple of spare hours and an appointment.

Not all hair extensions are the same, so make sure you choose the right ones for your hair. People with fine hair usually opt for 'stick-in' extensions, which are glued to the roots of your own hair. While these pump up your volume in a big way, there is a long-term downside to this method: added weight can cause the hair to snap, so you can end up with less than you started with. Everyday tasks like washing your hair become somewhat difficult, so it is only worth opting for these extensions if you are prepared to maintain them with regular salon visits. If your hair is reasonably thick, weaving may be the best answer. Strands of hair are woven into your own tresses. You do not have the waxy joins of 'stick-ins', and they are easy to weave out again.

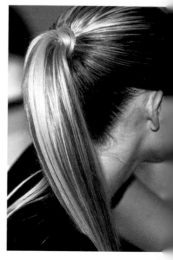

FAKING IT?

1 Make sure you choose a reputable salon. Listen to word of mouth.

2 Do not rush into it. Try on a wig of the same length that you are contemplating before you take the plunge – this will help you make sure the hairstyle suits you before it is too late.

3 Go for it: hair extensions do not have to be subtle. Experiment with brightly coloured hairpieces for a bold, modern look.

4 Remember that, like a dog, hair extensions are not just for Christmas. They require time and dedication, and look good only if you make the effort to maintain them.

5 Once hair extensions are in place, treat them as you would your own locks, but with a slightly lighter touch.

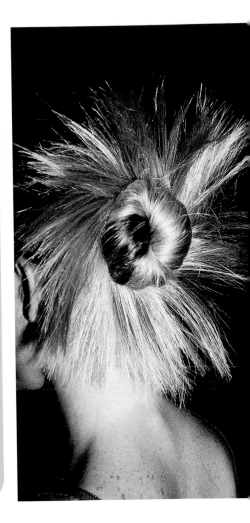

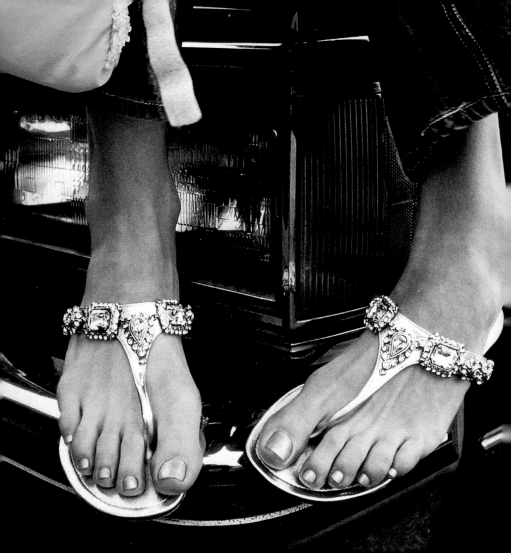

8 manicure & pedicure

'Every woman can have beautiful and healthy nails.'
Jessica Vartoughian, manicurist to the stars

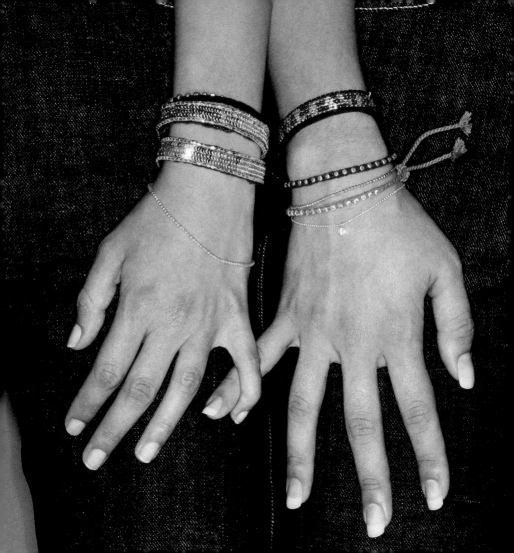

manicure

Hands up if you have regular manicures? Believe it or not, until recently, British women did not dedicate even a quarter of the time they spent cleansing, toning and moisturizing their faces to caring for their hands. Having manicures was left to our chic French counterparts, whose 'French manicure' has become the international 'no make-up' of nail care, and the Americans, who have nail bars on every street in New York. Not so any more. Thanks to fashion's new interest in our extremities (designers send models down the runway sporting anything from barbed-wire spokes to diamanté fingernails), more and more women have latched onto the trend for speaking volumes through their fingers. No longer content with a single layer of transparent varnish, we change the shape and colour of our nails with as much gusto as we change our kitten heels and snakeskin handbags. 'These days women enjoy experimenting with streaks and multicoloured effects,' says Susie Fitouri, a manicurist at Alexander McQueen's shows. 'Blue, black and yellow are no longer the domain of the outlandish – normal women paint their nails these colours, too.'

Texture, the modern buzz word of make-up, has found its way into nail care as well. Nail art and jewellery, not to mention sparkling glitter polishes, lend a 3-D aspect to otherwise ordinary nails. What's more, thanks to nail technology, you no longer have to be genetically programmed to achieve a beautiful set of fingernails.

HANDCARE

1 Invest in a water softener. Washing your hands in soft water makes a radical difference to their condition.

2 Treat your hands with a mild body exfoliator about once a week. This will encourage desquamation (the shedding of old skin cells) and the formation of new cells and smooth skin.

3 Use a hand cream with SPF. Carry a tube in your handbag and reapply it every time you wash your hands.

4 Ensure that you protect your nails as well as your skin from the sun. Always use a top coat with sun protection filters.

5 If you have discoloured nail beds, use diluted denture cleansing tablets and a nailbrush to scrub your fingertips. This bleaches unsightly stains, but go gently so that you do not tear the cuticles.

6 Never, ever cut your cuticles. They are there to protect your nails against bacteria. Instead, massage in cuticle cream, petroleum jelly or warm almond oil before you go to bed, and push your cuticles back gently when they are still warm and wet after a shower.

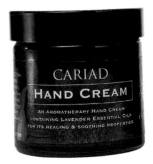

7 Use ridge filler to even out bumps in your nails (avoid pearlized varnish, as this highlights the problem).

8 Remember that a French manicure looks great even on really short nails.

9 Invest in a proper base coat (this feels slightly tacky even after it has dried and helps 'stick' the nail colour on) and a top coat (which dries hard and seals in the colour).

10 If treating yourself to a do-it-yourself manicure, file your fingernails before you remove old varnish. This will protect them during filing and prevent them from splitting.

11 Avoid filing nails into a point. Squarish edges and a slightly rounded middle are far more flattering.

12 Choose a nail varnish that complements your skin tone. If you have blue-toned skin, use cool nail varnishes like reds and pinks.

13 Make use of your scented candles. Once a pool of wax has formed, blow out the flame and let it cool. Then dip your fingers in the warm wax and rub it into your cuticles. It will condition the skin in the same way as a professional paraffin-wax treatment.

14 Wear gloves in cold weather to protect your hands from the wind and to stop your skin from dehydrating and flaking.

TOOLS OF THE TRADE

If you want to reap the benefits of beautifully manicured fingers, you must be prepared to put in the necessary time and effort. Have the right tools handy and you will be well on the way to a polished set of digits.

SHARP NAIL SCISSORS
The sharper your nail scissors, the cleaner the cut and the less likely you are to chip your nails. Buy a pair with slightly curved edges, as these create a more natural line when you are cutting.

NAIL BUFFER
This looks and acts much like a nailfile, although its surfaces are far smoother. Rub it over your nail beds using even motions to create a smoother surface and a gleaming finish.

NAILFILE
Once the simple emery board with its coarse surfaces was the only way to file your nails. Luckily, files today are far more refined – they leave nail edges smooth and velvety to the touch.

CUTICLE CREAM
Cuticles should be softened and pushed back, not cut. Some cuticle creams contain alpha-hydroxy acids (AHAs), which help remove surface skin cells and stop cuticles thickening.

HAND CREAM

Some hand creams are now so sophisticated that they contain bleaching agents to help reduce giveaway signs of ageing such as liver spots. Make sure that you always use a hand cream containing SPF. If you do not want to invest in a separate hand cream, remember that what is good enough for your face is certainly good enough for your fingers. Simply rub any leftover facial moisturizer into your hands.

THINGS TO AVOID

1 'Avoid nail hardeners if you have brittle nails,' says top London manicurist Iris Chapple. 'People with weak nails often think that their nails need hardening, when in reality they are already too dry, and need softening instead.'

2 Do not use clippers on fingernails. These are intended for harder toenails, give too square a finish and can encourage breakage.

3 Stay away from nail varnish removers containing acetone (unless you are doing a top-speed manicure – see page 308), as they will dry out the nail bed.

4 Remember that the most expensive is not necessarily the best. According to Professor Christopher Griffiths of the dermatology department at England's University of Manchester, 'Buying very expensive hand cream usually means that you are spending more on packaging. Cheaper products do just as much good, as the best products are ointments (water-based creams evaporate too quickly) which lock moisture in.'

COTTON OR MUSLIN HANDKERCHIEF

This should be used to push back the cuticles after you have had a warm shower.

RIDGE FILLER

This is a resin that helps smooth over uneven surfaces before you apply polish.

ALMOND OIL

If you want to turbo-condition your nails, rub almond oil into your cuticles before you go to bed. It keeps the skin soft and strengthens the nail bed, and encourages the growth of stronger, harder nails.

ACETONE-FREE NAIL VARNISH REMOVER

This formula will help to keep your nails moisturized, as well as removing any traces of unwanted colour.

BASE COAT AND TOP COAT

Although both these types of varnish are transparent, they perform very different functions. The base coat is moisturizing and remains slightly tacky to the touch, which helps it stick varnish onto the nail bed. The top coat, meanwhile, dries very quickly and locks colour in place. It is too drying to be used directly on the nail itself.

NAIL FACTS

1 Your nails grow about 1 mm (½ in) a week, which is quite a lot when you consider an entire nail is only 1 cm (¹⁄₁₆ in) or so long.

2 Poor diet affects nail growth – white spots may indicate a lack of calcium, so go easy on those fat-free diets if you want long nails.

3 An entire nail renews itself every 3–4 months.

POLISH TEXTURES

Nail varnish is no longer the straightforward brush'n'lacquer product it once was. Today, texture, as much as colour, plays a part in deciding exactly which polish is right for which occasion.

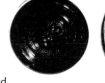
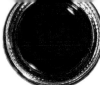

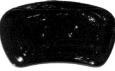

1 Traditional nail lacquer is best applied in two coats. It dries with a glossy finish and is available in plain, pearlized and glittery shades.

2 Fast-drying nail lacquer is great if you are in a hurry. These fast-drying polishes take only moments to dry, but do not have the same glossy finish as traditional varnish.

3 Polish pens are very convenient for carrying round in your bag for emergency touch-ups. These polishes work like felt-tip pens for easy application.

4 Peel-off polishes are something of a gimmick. These nail colours tend to be very thick and start bubbling and lifting before you want to remove them. While they do make nail varnish remover redundant, they have not really reached a level in quality that makes them any competition to a traditional varnish.

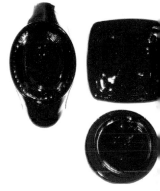

THE PERFECT MANICURE IN MINUTES

1 To strengthen your nails, brush them with a soft nailbrush while you are in the bath or shower. This will boost the circulation and encourage your nails to grow better.

2 Next, treat yourself to a cuticle cream, which will soften the skin and dissolve any dead skin cells that have accumulated. Gently push back the cuticles with a damp handkerchief or a muslin square.

3 Using a cotton wool pad, remove your old nail varnish by wiping your nails with a nail varnish remover that contains acetone. This will slightly dehydrate your nails and should therefore only be used if you are really pushed for time, but it will help the nail varnish fix more firmly onto the nails.

4 Save time by clipping your nails to remove excess length, and then smoothing off the edges with a file, always filing in one direction only.

5 Use a base coat followed directly by a top coat. These products dry more quickly than coloured nail varnishes and will leave your hands with a healthy shine and an overall groomed look.

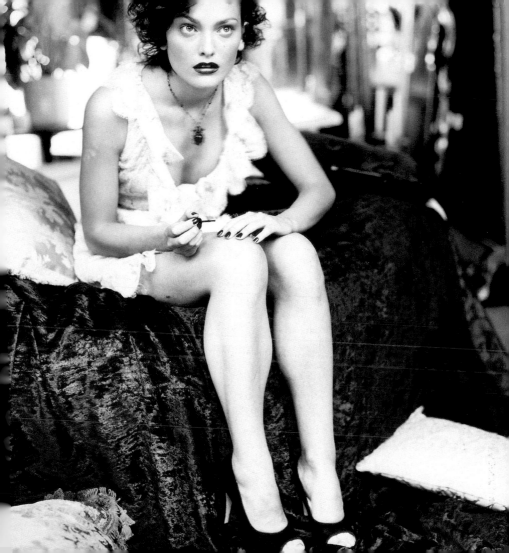

THE PERFECT POLISH

1 Gently buff your nails to smooth out any uneven surfaces.

2 Apply a thin layer of base coat to your nails. Allow it to dry for at least a minute before applying coloured varnish.

3 Next, turn your coloured varnish upside down once, then roll the bottle between your palms. This will ensure that the texture is even. Never shake your nail varnish upside down, as this upsets the balance of the colour pigments.

4 Apply varnish to each nail using three even brushstrokes. First colour the middle of the nail, and then fill in the stripes on either side. Always leave a small gap by the cuticle.

5 Finally, coat your nails in a fast-drying top coat, which will ensure they are touch dry within a couple of minutes and also acts as a sealant. As with the coloured varnish, avoid letting the top coat touch your cuticles, as it will cause them to dry out and flake.

6 When your nails are touch dry, dip your hands in a bowl of cold water to help set the varnish. Do not hold your fingers under a tap (faucet) of cold running water, as the water pressure will make the varnish slide.

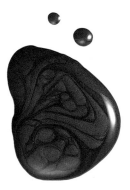

THE NATURAL MANICURE

According to Goro Uesugi, manicurist to half of Hollywood (including Winona Ryder and Angelica Houston), 'Nails are like hair. If you keep them clean, they will look better.'

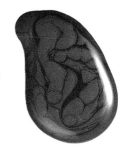

1 Uesugi suggests adding a couple of drops of bath oil to a bowl of hot water to soften your cuticles, before using a cotton bud (Q-Tip) dipped in cuticle remover to remove any protruding skin.

2 Cut your nails, using just a single cutting movement, to create a squarish shape. File the edges gently, always using the nailfile in the same direction and employing short, broken movements, as opposed to a 'sawing' technique.

3 Next, wash your fingertips in soapy water. This works better than varnish remover to create a clean surface, as it is not so drying.

4 Dry your fingertips, and add one coat of clear base coat to each nail.

5 Next, apply one coat only of a pale pinky-peach nail varnish. The single coat adds just a hint of colour, without being thick enough to look opaque. Essie's Ballet Slippers is my favourite for achieving this natural look.

6 Finish off the manicure with just a single layer of top coat.

THE FRENCH MANICURE

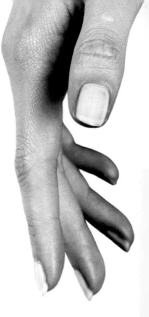

Great for day-through-to-evening wear, the French manicure has become an international favourite, as it leaves even the shortest nails looking great.

1 To create a French manicure, begin by preparing the hands and shaping the nails in the usual way (see page 308).

2 Apply a base coat to clean, dry nails (see page 308).

3 This is where manicurists vary:

OPTION 1: Apply the opaque white tip polish which has made this manicure famous straight away. This way, it is easy to even up any wobbly lines with a cotton bud (Q-Tip) dipped in a little nail varnish remover. Once the tips are satisfactory, follow up with two coats of a pale pink or peach varnish. Lastly, cover in top coat.

OPTION 2: Apply one coat of the peachy or pink colour to the entire nail bed. Next, apply the opaque white tip – using this method, you have to make certain that you get it right first time. When this has dried, apply a second coat of the coloured varnish, which in effect 'sandwiches' in the white tip. Lastly, apply your top coat.

THE AMERICAN MANICURE

Exactly the same procedure is involved in the American manicure as the French manicure, but a natural-coloured clear varnish is employed instead of the pinky or peach colour used in the European version. This makes the nail tips stand out far more than in the French manicure.

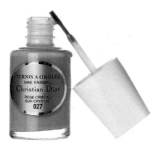

TRENDY NAILS

1 The fashion for piercing has reached every extremity, including one's nails. Unless you have super-strong talons, it is best to wear a ready-pierced false nail. Anything from mini rings to diamanté studs can be found. If piercing is not for you, a diamanté bindi looks just as good.

2 The trend for painting nails in contrasting colours, or with stars, hearts or flowers, was originated by Afro-Caribbean Americans. The style was picked up on the catwalk and has now filtered down to street level.

3 Mehndi designs look spectacular when applied to hands and nails. Give your nails a full manicure and then wait for at least 15 minutes. using a sharp white eyeliner, trace your chosen design along your little finger and down the side of your hand, ending up at the base of your wrist. Trace over the design using a fine-tipped brush dipped in body paint.

4 Diamanté jewels on the fingernails add a touch of modern glamour to any look. Before applying the top coat of your chosen nail varnish stick one self-adhesive bindi to the tip of each nail. Ensure you apply each bindi in the same spot on each nail. Jewels tend to work best for eveningwear, as they reflect light and look more dressy. Paint your top coat over the bindis and allow to dry.

MOST GIRLS FAKE IT

Who is to know that Mother Nature did not bless you with a perfect set of talons? Thanks to today's techniques and advances in technology, you can now mend unwanted splits, increase the length of your natural nails or sport a whole set of falsies that still look entirely natural. So go on, get your claws out ...

GEL EXTENSIONS

These are the modern way to improve your nails and are available at most good salons. First, the nails are buffed, before false nails are glued to the middle of the real nail. The nails are then buffed once again to get rid of any unwanted ridges. Once the nails are smooth, the therapist cuts and shapes the gel extension just as though it were a natural nail, and gel is applied to the entire length of the nail. Finally, the client places her hands under an ultraviolet light for approximately 5 minutes to allow her nails to harden.

'The great thing about gel extensions,' says top London manicurist Debra Poluck, 'is that they are not as much of an irritant as some of the previous extension methods and tend to cause less allergic reactions than the more traditional acrylic nail.'

FIBREGLASS

This can be used alone to increase your natural length, or in conjunction with a false nail. First, the nails are buffed, so that they are smooth and clean. Next, fibreglass strips are placed along the whole nail, glued down with nail glue, and cut or filed into shape. Fibreglass tips help protect your nails and allow them to grow without breaking. They also make polish last longer. Alternatively, a false nail can be applied (again to the middle of the natural nail), then covered in fibreglass strips, which are in turn buffed to ensure an even finish and then shaped. Once they are dry, polish is applied as usual.

ACRYLIC NAILS

These are the longest lasting of the falsies, but they can cause allergic reactions so always test out one nail before you invest in a whole set. First, the nails are buffed as usual to ensure a clean, dry surface. A false nail is then glued to the middle of the natural nail. Once the glue has dried, the nails are buffed again to make sure there are no ridges. The nails are then filed into shape. Next, an acrylic paste is mixed and, once it has reached an even consistency, it is painted over the whole nail. After it has dried for a few minutes, the manicurist will buff, smooth, shine and apply polish. Acrylic nails are between three and six times stronger than your natural nails and are the longest lasting of the false nail family.

SILK WRAPPING

This is a great strengthening treatment for nails that split easily or a rescue remedy for a single broken nail. It involves a layer of silk being glued to the nail and the rough edges being buffed.

NAIL PATCHES

These work much like plasters (adhesive strips), by sticking two sides of a split nail back together. They are best cut to size and applied in a professional salon, rather than at home.

BIO-SCULPTURE

The newest form of nail extension, bio-sculpture is the first system to use a single 'gel varnish' to extend the nails. The varnish is painted on, then set under an ultraviolet light. Once set, the nail is filed into shape. As the nail grows out, more varnish can be used to fill in the gap at the cuticle.

HOW TO BE A CONVINCING FAKER

Only wear false nails for a couple of weeks at a time to avoid infections developing. Always allow your nails a few days' respite between applications. If your nail beds start to look yellowish, see a pharmacist or a doctor in case you have developed an infection.

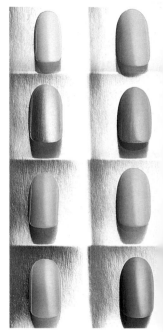

glorious feet

Believe it or not, the feet are the most erogenous zone of the body – surprising, perhaps, when you consider that they contain more sweat glands than any other part of our anatomy, so looking after our feet should be as natural to us as cleansing our faces.

HOME CARE

BARE FACTS

Kicking your shoes off helps to boost the condition of your feet enormously, as it frees the bones from the constraints of pointy shoes. The most effective way to rid yourself of soft corns is to walk barefoot as much as possible.

RELAX

Your feet often have to bear twice your body's weight. It is therefore vital to relieve them of the pressure occasionally. A bowl of hot water, reeking deliciously of aromatherapy oils, is a great way to lighten the load – soak your feet at least once a week for maximum effect. (Essential oils penetrate the bloodstream – use lavender for relaxing, peppermint for cooling down or eucalyptus for its antiseptic properties. Avoid using essential oils if you are pregnant.)

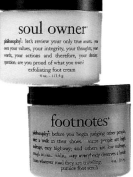

soul owner
philosophy: let's review your only true assets. you
own your values, your integrity, your thoughts, your
work, your actions and therefore, your desire.
question: are you proud of what you own?
exfoliating foot cream
4 oz. – 113.4 g.

footnotes
philosophy: before you begin judging other people,
take a walk in their shoes. some people are high-
mileage, easy highway; and others are low mileage,
rough terrain. either way everybody deserves a break
from whatever road they are traveling.   4 oz. – 113.4 g.
pumice foot scrub

BE A SOFTIE

Hard skin is not only uncomfortable, but also unsightly. The most effective way to remove it is over time with a pumice stone. Never tackle hard skin with a razor, as you can bet your bottom dollar you will cut yourself. A foot file, used on a nightly basis, will ensure you don't end up with a pair of trotters encased in hard skin.

PUT YOUR BEST FOOT FORWARD

Fashion decrees that toenails be cut straight across (preferably with a toenail clipper), rather than rounded at the edges. This will ensure that your look is up to date and protect your nail beds as you walk. Rub warm almond oil into your cuticles to keep them in peak condition, and don't be afraid to slather body moisturizer from head to toe as part of the quest for perfect feet.

POLISH UP YOUR ACT

Before painting your little piggies, separate them with cotton wool to prevent the varnish from smudging. In most cases, dark, vibrant colours look best on toes. For a holiday treat, though, a French polish (pale pink with white tips – see page 312) works wonders with a tan.

FEET TREATS

1 Paraffin-wax treatments, which are fabulously moisturizing for the cuticles and surrounding skin, can be used on hands and feet. They usually involve sealing the chosen area in warm, wet wax and letting it set, before prizing open the wax and finishing off with a massage.

2 Regular exfoliation keeps feet looking young. Invest in a body scrub (Clinique and Chanel make my favourites), and spend a few minutes a week working all over the feet, using repeated, circular motions on any areas of hard skin. A pumice stone will help remove any stubborn patches.

3 Use a nailbrush to push back the cuticles on your toenails during a bath or shower. As with your hands, never cut overgrown cuticles.

4 Remember that filing your toenails into pointed shapes can lead to the pain of ingrowing toenails and infections. Always clip your toenails straight across.

5 For sweet-smelling feet, rub the soles with surgical spirit.

6 Massage your own feet. Even if you are not adept in the art of reflexology, a little aromatherapy oil, kneaded from the soles of the feet upwards toward the knee, is a great way to relax and take the stress off your tired feet.

7 A top treat for feet is to slather your feet with Vaseline and put on cotton socks before you go to bed, then go to sleep. The heat generated in the socks will double the softening properties of the Vaseline, and you will wake up with baby soft feet.

TOE TREATS

PUMICE STONE is the best foot file. Wet the grey stone, rub some soap into it and file away at unsightly lumps of hard skin. Or splash out on a Diamancel Foot File. Although it is very expensive, it is worth the investment as it lasts a lifetime. The real diamond chips contained in the file will stop removing skin once they touch the moist new skin underneath.

REPAIR CREAM from the Institut de Jambes, which is specifically devoted to leg and foot care, is a wonderful cream that moisturizes dry legs; its menthol base is a great pick-me-up for tired feet. Treat yourself to some next time you are in Paris.

LAIT JAMBES LOURDES by Clarins is a cooling lotion which looks and smells minty. It can be applied over tights (panty hose), to relieve your legs when you don't have time to go home and put your feet up.

PEPPERMINT FOOT LOTION from the Body Shop is hard to beat for price and results.

REFLEXOLOGY is based on the philosophy that energy channels that pass through every organ of the body end in the feet. By massaging specific areas of the feet, practitioners work on corresponding areas of the body. Complaints such as back ache, migraines, PMT, eczema, acne and psoriasis can all be helped – usually when traditional medicine has proved unsatisfactory.

CLASSIC RED

1 First, apply cuticle cream to your toenails, then soak your feet in a bowl of steaming, soapy water to soften any hard skin.

2 Push back your cuticles with a damp face cloth or handkerchief, and gently file away any patches of hard skin. Stop filing as soon as the moist new skin appears.

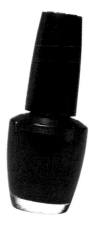

3 Clip your toenails with a toenail clipper, using a straight-across motion. Cut them so that the tip of the toe itself is slightly visible beyond the edge of the nail. File the edges gently with a nailfile, making sure not to remove the square edges.

4 Next, remove any traces of old nail varnish using a non-acetone nail varnish remover, which will not dry out the nails. (The old varnish will protect the toes during filing, so do not remove it until this point.)

5 Separate your toes using pieces of cotton wool to prevent individual nails from smudging.

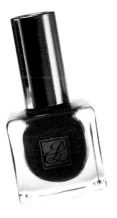

6 Apply your base coat evenly over each nail. This will help protect the nail.

7 Allow the base coat a few moments to dry, then apply two coats of bright red varnish (YSL's Rouge Pur No. 11 is my

preferred choice). First, apply a single, continuous straight line up the middle of the toenail, starting just above the cuticle and ending at the tip. Next, apply one continuous line to the left and one to the right of the central colour strip, leaving a small gap at either side of the toenail for a professional-looking finish.

8 Apply a second coat of red varnish in exactly the same way as the first coat.

9 Finally, after allowing the varnish a few minutes' drying time, apply a top coat.

10 Avoid wearing shoes for 20 minutes at least. When you do, try to wear sandals that do not cover the toes. Do not wear tights (panty hose) or socks for at least an hour or all your hard work will be ruined.

BEACH FEET

This French manicure is fabulous for the beach, as it complements a tan perfectly. As a bonus, it also goes with clothes of any colour from black to fuchsia.

1 First soak your feet in steaming, soapy water to soften any hard skin.

2 Treat your cuticles and file any hard skin in exactly the same way as instructed on page 321.

3 Next, clip your toenails, leaving them fractionally longer than you would do for the 'Classic Red' pedicure. (The tip of the toe should be in line with the end of your toenail for this pedicure.) You can also use a toenail clipper to remove any bits of overhanging skin, which tend to start growing either side of the little toenails.

4 Remove old varnish with a non-acetone varnish remover.

5 Next, part your toes with cotton wool, and apply a single, clear base coat.

6 Using a French manicure kit, apply one coat of the pink/ peachy colour over your toes, using the 'three-stripe' technique described opposite.

7 Once this coat is completely dry, very carefully apply the opaque white varnish in one continuous straight line across the tip of each toe. It is easier to apply this neatly to your toenails than to your own fingernails.

8 Once again, wait until this is absolutely dry (to avoid smudging), before applying a second coat of the peachy/ pink colour to each toenail.

9 Finally, apply a clear top coat.

MEHNDI FEET

1 Prepare your feet in the same way as always, up to and including separating your toes with cotton wool.

2 Next, take your mehndi mixture, which should be prepared 24 hours in advance. First, make the paste by mixing a staining agent with 2 teaspoons instant coffee powder. Microwave the paste on high for 20 seconds and then allow it to cool. Next, put 1 heaped tablespoon henna powder into a bowl, and add the prepared paste bit by bit, stirring until it reaches the smooth consistency of toothpaste.

3 Using a white eyeliner pencil, draw a design along the outer edge of the foot, swirling up towards the toes. Flowers work particularly well on feet, as do simple, geometric designs.

4 When you are happy with the design, use a very fine-tipped brush to trace carefully over the white pattern with the henna mixture. Keep the line fairly thin so that it does not smudge.

5 After it has dried, set the design with lemon juice (allow it to dry on the foot), then apply your varnish as always – deep brown, burgundy and bronze look best with henna.

6 For a bindi pedicure, just varnish your toes as always, and apply bindi stickers to your toenails (in exactly the same position on each toe). Apply top coat over the bindi sticker to give it extra staying power.

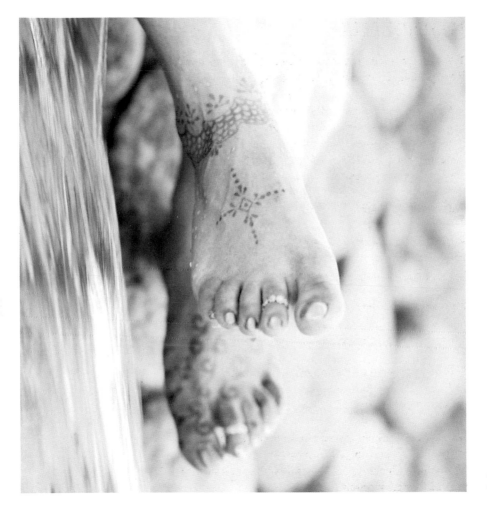

DIRECTORY

uk

make-up

COSMETICS À LA CARTE LTD
19b Motcomb Street
London SW1 8LB
Tel: 020 7235 0696
www.a-la-carte.co.uk

FARMACIA
Tel: 020 7637 5827
www.farmacia123.com

HARVEY NICHOLS
109–25 Knightsbridge
London SW1X 7RJ
Tel: 020 7235 5000
www.harveynichols.com

HOUSE OF FRASER
Head Office
1 Howick Place
London SW1P 1BH
Tel: 020 7963 2000
www.houseoffraser.co.uk

JOHNNY LOVES ROSIE
Tel: 020 7375 3574
www.johnnylovesrosie.
co.uk

LIBERTY
210–220 Regent Street
London W1B 5AH
Tel: 020 7734 1234
www.liberty.co.uk

MOLTON BROWN COSMETICS
58 South Molton Street
London W1K 5SL
Tel: 020 7499 6474
www.moltonbrown.co.uk

POUT
32 Shelton Street
London WC2H 9JE
Tel: 020 7379 0379
www.pout.co.uk

SCREEN FACE
48 Monmouth Street
London WC2 9EP
Tel: 020 7836 3955
www.screenface.com

SELFRIDGES
400 Oxford Street
London W1A 2LR
Tel: 0800 123 400
www.selfridges.com

SEPHORA
Brent Cross Shopping
Centre
London, NW4 3FP
Tel: 020 8457 9445
www.sephora.com

SHU UEMURA
24 Neal Street
London WC2H 9QW
Tel: 020 7240 7635
www.shuuemura.com

SPACE NK
www.spacenk.co.uk

skincare & spas

ALLERGENICS
For stockists call:
01274 526 360
www.optimah.com

AMANDA LACEY
Tel: 020 7351 4443
www.amandalacey.com
Facialist with product range

**ATHENAEUM HOTEL
AND APARTMENTS**
116 Piccadilly
London W1J 7BJ
Tel: 020 7499 3464
www.athenaeumhotel.com
Great spa treatments

BALANCE
250 King's Road
London SW3 5UE
Tel: 020 7565 0333
www.balancetheclinic.com

**THE BERKELEY HEALTH
CLUB AND SPA**
The Berkeley
Wilton Place
Knightsbridge
London SW1X 7RL
Tel: 020 7235 6000
www.the-berkeley.co.uk
Fabulous spa facilities

**BHARTI VYAS HOLISTIC
THERAPY & BEAUTY CENTRE**
5 & 24 Chiltern Street
London W1U 7QE
Tel: 020 7935 5312
www.bharti-vyas.com

CLARINS
For stockists and salons
call: 020 7307 6700
www.uk.clarins.com

DARPHIN
www.darphin.com

DECLEOR
For approved locations
call: 020 7313 8780
www.decleor.co.uk
Essential oil-based skincare

**NOELLA GABRIELLE,
AROMATHERAPIST
AT ELEMIS**
The Lodge
92 Uxbridge Road
Harrow Weald
Middlesex HA3 6DQ
For mail order, product or
salon and spa enquiries
call: 01278 727830
www.elemis.com

ENVIRON
For stockists and salons
call: 020 8450 2020
www.environ.co.za

EUPHORIA
29 Elystan Street
London SW3 3NT
Tel: 020 7584 3344

EVE LOM
2 Spanish Place
London W1U 3HU
Tel: 020 7935 9988
www.evelom.co.uk
Facialist with product range

GATINEAU
For stockists and mail
order call:
freephone 0800 731 5805;
for salons call: 01753
620 881

GUINOT
For stockists and salons
call: 01344 873 123

**FARIDA CHOUDHURY, FOR
BROW SHAPING AT URBAN
RETREAT AT HARRODS**
Knightsbridge
London SW1X 7XL
Tel: 020 7893 8333
www.urbanretreat.co.uk

JURLIQUE
Australian natural
skincare and
aromatherapy
Tel: 08707 700980
www.jurlique.com.au

LA PRAIRIE
www.laprairie.com

**VAISHALY PATEL AT
MARTYN MAXEY**
18 Grosvenor Street
London W1X 9FD
Tel: 020 7629 6161
www.martynmaxey.co.uk

**JUDY NAAKE FOR ST TROPEZ
FAKE TANNING**
www.st-tropez.co.uk

NORMA NEWMAN
154 King's Road
London SW6 4LZ
Tel: 020 7731 2323
*Facials, manicures, pedicures,
waxing and massage*

THE RUNNYMEDE HOTEL
Windsor Road, Egham
Surrey TW20 0AG
Tel: 01784 436 171
www.runnymedehotel.com
*Huge pool and every spa
treatment under the sun*

SOPHIE THORPE
106 Draycott Avenue
Chelsea
London SW3 3AE
Tel: 020 7589 5899
*Eyebrow tattooing, Environ
and Darphin facials and
manicures*

manicures & pedicures

IRIS CHAPPLE
3 Spanish Place
London W1U 3XH
Tel: 020 7486 6001

NAILS INC
41 South Molton Street
London W1Y 1HB
Tel: 020 7499 8333
www.nailsinc.com

hair salons

AVEDA CONCEPT SALON
Harvey Nichols
Knightsbridge
London SW1X 7RJ
Tel: 020 7201 8610
www.aveda.co.uk
*Antoinet Beenders for
styling*

THE AVEDA INSTITUTE
174 High Holborn
Covent Garden
London WC1V 7AA
Tel: 020 7759 7355
www.aveda.co.uk

CHARLES WORTHINGTON
7 Percy Street
London W1T 1DH
Tel: 020 7631 1370
www.charlesworthington.
co.uk

DANIEL GALVIN
58–60 George Street
London W1U 7ET
Tel: 020 7486 96611
www.daniel-galvin.co.uk

**LUKE HERSHESON AT
DANIEL HERSHESON**
45 Conduit Street
London W1S 2YN
Tel: 020 7434 1747
www.danielhersheson.
co.uk

HUGH AND STEPHEN
161 Ebury Street
London SW1W 9QN
Tel: 020 7730 2196

ERROL DOUGLAS
18 Motcomb Street
London SW1X 8LB
Tel: 020 7235 0110
www.erroldouglas.com

JO HANSFORD
19 Mount Street
London W1K 2RN
Tel: 020 7495 7774
www.johansford.com

JOHN FRIEDA
4 Aldford Street
London W1K 2AE
Tel: 020 7491 0840
www.johnfrieda.co.uk

DEREK THOMPSON AT
MICHAELJOHN
25 Albemarle Street
London W15 4HU
Tel: 020 7629 6969
www.michaeljohn.co.uk

FRANCES VAN CLARKE AT
MICHAEL VAN CLARKE
1 Beaumont Street
London W1G 6DF
Tel: 020 7224 3123
www.vanclarke.com

NICKY CLARKE
130 Mount Street
London W1K 3NY
Tel: 084488 48888
www.nickyclarke.com

REAL
8 Cale Street
Chelsea Green
London SW3 3QU
Tel: 020 7589 0877
www.realhair.co.uk

TONI AND GUY
www.toniandguy.co.uk

TREVOR SORBIE
27 Floral Street
London WC2E 9DP
Tel: 020 7379 6901
www.trevorsorbie.com

UMBERTO GIANNINI
www.umbertogiannini.
co.uk

WINDLE
41 Shorts Gardens
London WC2H 9AP
Tel: 020 7497 2393

specialist treatments & organizations

THE AROMATHERAPY
ORGANIZATIONS COUNCIL
PO Box 19834
London SE25 6WF
Tel: 020 8251 7912
www.aromatherapy-uk.org

THE BRITISH ASSOCIATION
OF AESTHETIC SURGEONS
35–43 Lincoln's Inn Fields
London WC2A 3PE
Tel: 020 7405 2234
www.baaps.co.uk

THE BRITISH ASSOCIATION
OF DERMATOLOGISTS
4 Fitzroy Square
London W1T 5HQ
Tel: 020 7383 0266
www.bad.org.uk

THE BRITISH COSMETIC
SURGERY ADVISORY BUREAU
Tel: 0800 013 6723

BRITISH INSTITUTE
AND ASSOCIATION OF
ELECTROLYSIS
Tel: 0870 128 0477
www.electrolysis.co.uk

THE INSTITUTE OF
OPTIMUM NUTRITION
Avalon House 72
Lower Mortlake Road
Richmond
Surrey TW9 2JY
Tel: 020 8614 7800
www.ion.ac.uk

JANE CLARKE CONSULTANCY
29–30 Frith Street
London W1J 5TL
Tel: 020 7437 3767
Nutritionist

WENDY LEWIS
Tel: 001 212 861 6148
www.wlbeauty.com
Cosmetic surgery consultant

NICHOLAS LOWE
Cranley Clinic
Harcourt House
Cavendish Square
London W1G 0PN
Tel: 020 7499 3223
Botox and dermatology

DR ANDREW MARKEY
Consultant Dermatologist
at St John's Institute of
Dermatology, St Thomas's
Hospital, and privately at
The Lister Hospital
Chelsea Bridge Road
London SW1W 8RH
Tel: 020 7730 1219
info@lister.hcahealthcare.
co.uk

DR JEAN-LOUIS SEBAGH
25 Wimpole Street
London W1M 7AD
Tel: 020 7637 0548
doctor@frenchcosmetic.
com
Botox and liposuction

THE SOCIETY OF
CHIROPODISTS AND
PODIATRISTS
1 Fellmonger's Path
Tower Bridge Road
London SE1 3LY
Tel: 020 7234 8620
www.feetforlife.org

usa

make-up

AVEDA
Tel: 866 823 1425
www.aveda.com

AVON
800/FOR AVON
www.avon.com
Retail and mail order
make-up and face care
products

BARNEYS NEW YORK
660 Madison Avenue
New York, NY 10021-8448
Tel: 212 826 8900
www.barneys.com

BENEFIT
Tel: 800 781 2336
www.benefitcosmetics.
com

BLOOMINGDALE'S
1000 3rd Avenue
New York, NY 10022
Tel: 800 777 4999
www.bloomingdales.com

BOBBI BROWN ESSENTIALS
Tel: 212 980 7040
www.bobbibrown
cosmetics.com

CALVIN KLEIN
Tel: 800 223 6808
www.calvinklein.com

CLINIQUE
Tel: 212 572 3800
www.clinique.com

ELIZABETH ARDEN
Tel: 1 866 217 2927
www.shop.elizabetharden.
com

ESTÉE LAUDER
www.esteelauder.com

LANCÔME
Tel: 800/LANCÔME
www.lancome-usa.com

REVLON
Tel: 800 473 8566
www.revlon.com

SEPHORA
Tel: 887 737 4672 for
branches worldwide
www.sephora.com

SHISEIDO
www.sca.shiseido.com
Skincare and cosmetics

SHU UEMURA
Tel: 1 888 748 5678
*Natural skincare and
cosmetics*

skincare & day spas

AVEDA SALON AND SPA
456 West Broadway
New York, NY 10012
Tel: 212 473 0280
www.aveda.com
*Professional facials, skincare
and make-up products*

BEAUTÉ DE PROVENCE
712 Fifth Avenue
Henri Bendel, Fourth Floor
New York, NY 10019
Tel: 212 753 9500
www.fredericfekkai.com
*Luxurious day spa offering
over 42 specialized
treatments including facials,
wraps, scrubs, massages,
pedicures and manicures*

BLISS SPA
568 Broadway
New York, NY 10012
Tel: 212 219 8970
www.blissworld.com
Treatments and skincare

DECLEOR USA
Tel: 888 414 4471
www.decleor.com

**ELIZABETH ARDEN RED DOOR
SALON AND SPA**
691 Fifth Avenue
New York, NY 10022
Tel: 212 546 0200
red.door@virgin.net
www.reddoorspas.com

GUINOT
Tel: 800 444 6621

Henri Bendel
Tel: 212 247 1100
www.henribendel.com

manicures & pedicures

ARSI SKINCARE
Suite 206 162 West 56th St
New York, NY 10022-1006
Tel: 212 582 5720

CELINA SALON
348 East 66th Street
New York, NY 10021-6830
Tel: 212 737 9500

hair salons

ART LUNA
8930 Keith Avenue
West Hollywood
Tel: 310 247 1383

FREDERIC FEKKAI
712 Fifth Avenue
Henri Bendel, Fourth Floor
New York, NY 10019
Tel: 212 753 9500
www.fredericfekkai.com

JOHN FRIEDA
30 East 76th Street
New York, NY 10021
Tel: 212 327 3400
www.johnfrieda.com

Louis Licari Salon
343 North Camden Drive
Beverly Hills, CA 90210
Tel: 310 247 0855
www.louislicari.com

Michaeljohn
414 North Camden Drive
Beverly Hills
CA 90210-4532
Tel: 310 278 8333

Salon Ishi
70 East 55th Street
New York, NY 10022
Tel: 212 888 4744
www.salonishi.com
*For an incredibly relaxing
scalp massage, ask for the
Shiatsu Shampoo*

Kris Sorbie
Global Artistic Director
for Colour, Redken
575 Fifth Avenue
New York, NY 10017
Tel: 212 984 4847

specialist
treatments
& organizations
**American Academy
of Facial Plastic and
Reconstructive Surgery**
310 S Henry Street
Alexandria, VA 22314
Tel: 703 299 9291
www.aafprs.org

**The American Board
of Dermatologists**
Henry Ford Health System
1 Ford Place
Detroit, MI 48202-3450
Tel: 313 874 1088
www.abderm.org

Skin treatment
advice and referrals
**The American Society
of Plastic Surgeons**
444 E Algonquin Road
Arlington Heights
IL 60005
Tel: 1 888 475 2784
www.plasticsurgery.org

**Bioelements Alpha-
Hydroxy
Acid Hotline**
Tel: 800 533 3064

websites

www.aveda.com
www.beautique.com
www.beauty.com
www.beautyscene.com
www.beautyspy.com
www.clinique.com
www.garden.co.uk
www.cosmetics.com
www.cosmeticscop.com
www.hairnet.com
www.cosmeticconnection.
com
www.lorealcosmetics.com
www.revlon.com

INDEX

picture credits

The publishers would like to thank the following sources for their kind permission to reproduce the pictures in this book:

All images © Vogue, The Condé Nast Publication Ltd, except where indicated.
t: top, b: bottom, l: left, r: right,
tl: top left, tr: top right, bl: bottom left, br: bottom right, bc: bottom centre, bcl: bottom centre left, bcr: bottom centre right

Miles Aldridge 143
Clive Arrowsmith 33
Enrique Badulescu 6, 44, 72, 76, 79
David Bailey 29, 31
Paul Bowden 157br, 174, 175, 200, 201, 202
Richard Burbridge 150, 160
Regan Cameron 98, 102, 141, 172, 177, 231, 248, 272, 297
Liz Collins 15
Paddy Cook 296b
Coopers 104
Sean Cunningham, 125, 135, 144br, 144bl, 148, 163, 166l, 169, 179, 184r, 184l, 185tr, 185br, 186tr, 186br, 189tr, 189br, 192, 195, 216l, 216r, 225, 228l, 228r, 240t, 240b, 251, 252, 253
Patrick Demarchelier 36,
Robin Derrick 1, 40, 43, 59,

61, 147, 187, 300
Matthew Donaldson 86, 87
Arthur Elgort 125, 309
Simon Emmett 188, 267, 318
Robert Erdmann 52, 54
Mary Evans Picture Library/ John Bettes 22
Fototheme 118, 119, 170, 171, 181br, 191, 207b, 209, 213, 215, 216, 221, 224t, 242, 292, 296t, 302
Ronald Grant Archive (Courtesy 20th Century Fox) 20
Horst 26
Kelly Klein 47, 133, 191, 255
Kobal Collection/ Paramount (Courtesy Kobal) Bud Fraker 28
Hiroshi Kutomi 206
Andrew Lamb 276
Peter Lindbergh 34
Wayne Maser 37, 38/39
Raymond Meier 16, 234, 258, 298
Tom Munro 88, 140, 183, 196, 227, 245
Norman Parkinson 32
Louisa Parry 307
Serge Paulet 112, 114, 115
Sudhir Pithwa 66, 108, 139, 142, 158, 162, 164, 180, 181t, 185bl, 189bl, 198, 207, 213, 214, 224b, 226, 229t, 229b, 230, 239, 250, 280, 285, 293, 310, 311, 313, 317, 321
Phil Poynter 101
Terry Richardson 80, 232,

263
Paolo Roversi 282
Thomas Schenk 121
David Slijper 70, 157, 222, 312
Vanina Sorrenti 12
Edward Steichen 25

The following images are copyright © Carlton Books Ltd.
Graham Atkins-Hughes 126
Lorraine Day 287, 325
Catherine Rowlands 281
Patrice de Villiers 4, 5, 9, 62, 102, 105, 111, 117, 123, 139, 144tr, 316

Every effort has been made to acknowledge correctly and contact the source and/ or copyright holder of each picture, and Carlton Books Limited apologizes for any unintentional errors or omissions which may be corrected in future editions of this book.

The publishers would like to thank the following companies, who kindly provided products for the photographic shoot. Alchemy, BeneFit Cosmetics, Bobbie Brown Essentials, Calvin Klein, Chantecaille, Chanel, Clinique, Debenhams, Elizabeth Arden, Estée Lauder, Fendi, Hard Candy Lancôme, Laura Mercier Lulu Guinness, Mister Mascara, MAC Cosmetics, Nars, Nuxe, Philosophy, Prada Beauty, Prescriptives Pupa, Ruby & Millie, Shu Uemura, Space NK, Stila Cosmetics, Tony & Tina, Tweezerman, Urban Decay and YSL

author credits

I would like to thank my family – Stuart, Anouska and my parents for all their love and support. I would also like to thank the many people who have helped with quotes and information for *Vogue Make-up*, Venetia Penfold for commissioning me and Kathy Phillips for giving me so many opportunities.